Whiplash Injury

Perspectives on the Development of Chronic Pain

Helge Kasch, MD, PhD

Dennis Turk, Professor, PhD

Troels S. Jensen, Professor, MD, DMSc

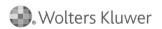 Wolters Kluwer

Philadelphia · Baltimore · New York · London
Buenos Aires · Hong Kong · Sydney · Tokyo

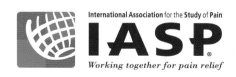

International Association for the Study of Pain

IASP

Working together for pain relief

Acquisitions Editor: Keith Donnellan
Product Development Editor: Nicole Dernoski
Editorial Assistant: Kathryn Leyendecker
Senior Production Project Manager: Alicia Jackson
Design Coordinator: Joan Wendt
Manufacturing Coordinator: Beth Welsh
Marketing Manager: Dan Dressler
Prepress Vendor: S4Carlisle Publishing Services

9 8 7 6 5 4 3 2 1

Printed in China

Library of Congress Cataloging-in-Publication Data

Names: Kasch, Helge, author. | Turk, Dennis C., author. | Jensen, Troels
   Staehelin, author.
Title: Whiplash injury : perspectives on the development of chronic pain /
   Helge Kasch, Dennis C. Turk, Troels S. Jensen.
Description: First edition. | Philadelphia : Wolters Kluwer Health, [2016] |
   Includes bibliographical references.
Identifiers: LCCN 2015028447 | ISBN 9781496333483
Subjects: | MESH: Whiplash Injuries--physiopathology. | Chronic
   Pain--etiology. | Whiplash Injuries--complications. | Whiplash
   Injuries--therapy.
Classification: LCC RD533.5 | NLM WE 708 | DDC 617.5/3044--dc23 LC record available at http://lccn.loc.gov/2015028447

LWW.com

Whiplash Injury

Perspectives on the Development of Chronic Pain

CONTRIBUTORS

Linda J. Carroll, PhD
Professor
School of Public Health
University of Alberta
Edmonton, Alberta

Tina Birgitte Wisbech Carstensen, PhD
Clinical Psychologist
Assistant Professor
The Research Clinic for Functional Disorders
  and Psychosomatics
Aarhus University Hospital
Aarhus, Denmark

Brian D. Corner, PhD
Research Anthropologist
Warfighter Directorate
US Army Natick Soldier RDEC
Natick, Massachusetts

James M. Elliott, PT, PhD
Assistant Professor
Department of Physical Therapy and Human
  Movement Sciences
Northwestern University
Feinberg School of Medicine
Chicago, Illinois
Honorary Senior Fellow
School of Health and Rehabilitation Sciences
University of Queensland
Queensland, Australia
Affiliate Professor
Zurich University of Applied Sciences
Zurich, Switzerland

Deborah Falla, BPhty (Hons), PhD
Professor
Pain Clinic
Center for Anesthesiology, Emergency and
  Intensive Care Medicine
University Hospital Gottingen
Department of Neurorehabilitation Engineering
Bernstein Focus Neurotechnology (BFNT)
  Bernstein Center for Computational
  Neuroscience
University Medical Center Gottingen
Georg-August University
Gottingen, Germany

Lisbeth Frostholm, PhD
Clinical Psychologist
Associate Professor
The Research Clinic for Functional Disorders
  and Psychosomatics
Aarhus University Hospital
Aarhus, Denmark

Meagan E. Ita, MS
Graduate Student
Department of Bioengineering
University of Pennsylvania
Philadelphia, Pennsylvania

Troels S. Jensen, MD, DMSc
Professor
Director IDNC,
Department of Neurology and
Danish Pain Research Center
Aarhus University Hospital
Aarhus, Denmark

Gwendolen Jull, MPhty, PhD, Grad Dip
Manip Ther Dip Phty FACP
Professor
Division of Physiotherapy
Director
NHMRC Center of Clinical Research
  Excellence in Spinal Pain, Injury
  and Health
Director
Cervical Spine and Whiplash
  Research Unit
University of Queensland
Queensland, Australia

Helge Kasch, MD, PhD
Associate Professor
Medical Research Director
Senior Consultant Neurologist
Research Department
Spinal Cord Injury Centre of
  Western Denmark
Department of Neurology
Regional Hospital of Viborg
Viborg, Denmark

Alice Kongsted, MSc (Clin Biomech), PhD
Chiropractor
Nordic Institute of Chiropractic and
   Clinical Biomechanics
Associate Professor
Department of Sports Science and Clinical
   Biomechanics
University of Southern Denmark
Odense, Denmark

Abhishek Kumar, BDS, PhD
Post Doctoral Fellow
Section Orofacial Pain and Jaw Function
Department of Dentistry
Faculty of Health
Aarhus University Hospital
Aarhus, Denmark
Department of Dental Medicine
Karolinska Institutet
Huddinge, Sweden
Also: member, Scandinavian Center for
   Orofacial Neurosciences (SCON)

Steven James Linton
Professor
Department of Clinical Psychology
Director
Center for Health and Medical Psychology
   (CHAMP)
Örebro University
Örebro, Sweden

Samuel A. McLean, MD, MPH
Attending Physician
Department of Emergency Medicine
Vice Chair, Research
Department of Anesthesiology
Associate Professor
Department of Emergency Medicine,
   Anesthesiology, and Psychiatry
University of North Carolina
Medical School Wing C,
Chapel Hill, North Carolina

James P. Robinson, MD, PhD
Professor
Department of Rehabilitation Medicine
University of Washington
UW Medicine Center for Pain Relief and
   the Bone and Joint Surgery Center
University of Washington
Seattle, Washington

Hans-George Schaible, MD
Professor
Institute of Physiology/Neurophysiology
Jena University Hospital
Jena, Germany

Brian D. Stemper, PhD
Associate Professor
Department of Neurosurgery
Medical College of Wisconsin
Research Biomedical Engineer, Research Service
Clement J. Zablocki Veterans Affairs Medical
   Center
Milwaukee, Wisconsin

*Michele Sterling, PhD, MPhty, BPhty, Grad
Dip Manip Physio, FACP*
Post Doctoral Fellow
NHMRC Centre of Research Excellence in
   Recovery Following Road Traffic Injuries
Associate Director
Centre of National Research on Disability and
   Rehabilitation Medicine (CONROD)
Menzies Health Institute Queensland
Griffith University
Parklands, Australia

Peter Svensson, DDS, PhD, Dr.Odont.
Professor and Head
Section Orofacial Pain and Jaw Function
Department of Dentistry
Faculty of Health
Aarhus University Hopsital
Aarhus, Denmark
Department of Dental Medicine
Karolinska Institutet
Huddinge, Sweden
Also: member, Scandinavian Center for
   Orofacial Neurosciences (SCON)

Dennis C. Turk, PhD
John and Emma Bonica Endowed Chair and
   Professor of Anesthesiology and Pain Research
Director
Center for Pain Research on Impact,
   Measurement, and Effectiveness (C-PRIME)
Department of Anesthesiology and Pain
   Medicine
University of Washington
Seattle, Washington

Fatemeh Vakilian, MSc
Doctoral Student
School of Public Health
University of Alberta
Edmonton, Canada

David M. Walton, PT, PhD, FCAMPT
Assistant Professor
School of Physical Therapy
Western University
Associate Scientist
Lawson Health Research Institute
Director
Pain and Quality of Life Integrated Research
    Lab Secretary
London, Canada

Beth A. Winkelstein, PhD
Bioengineer
Department of Bioengineering
School of Engineering and Applied Science
University of Pennsylvania
Philadelphia, Pennsylvania

PREFACE

SETTING THE SCENE

Neck injury, many cases of which are relatively mild, so-called whiplash injury, is commonly encountered following motor vehicle collisions. Although the primary presenting problem reported by those who report whiplash injuries is pain located in the neck, shoulder, and arm, along with headaches, widespread pain is also reported in some. In addition to physical symptoms, cognitive disturbances (i.e., problems of attention, concentration, and memory) and emotional distress may cause significant handicap and social disability in a proportion of these individuals, resulting in chronic pain and disability that may be very difficult to treat. Thus, even apparently minor collisions and cervical trauma may cause prolonged problems. Motor vehicle collisions and traumatic injuries to the neck therefore represent a significant health concern and are regarded as a major socioeconomic burden to society.

Currently, there is only limited knowledge to explain why certain patients recover from apparently minor head and neck injuries, while others develop persistent signs and symptoms. Available research suggests that a range of biological, social, and psychological factors are involved in eliciting and maintaining the pain and disability. Identification of significant risk factors at an early stage after injury is thus crucial in order to prevent and limit the transition from acute symptoms to chronic pain-related disability and improve treatment.

The intent of the 12th IASP Research Symposium convened in 2014 was to address the biopsychosocial factors involved in the development and course of chronic pain after whiplash, and to discuss whether whiplash injury might be a good model for the set of dysfunctional pain conditions. The organizers (HK, TSJ) were in contact with most of the invited speakers more than a year prior to the symposium. There was significant and shared enthusiasm for the importance of the topic.

A set of 22 international speakers spanning a wide array of research areas (e.g., biomechanics, anatomy, psychology, and clinical practice) were invited to the symposium, held at Aarhus University (Denmark) during March 21–23, 2014. Over one hundred delegates attended and participated in the 3-day meeting. Previous congresses held with a focus on whiplash injury have been characterized by significant and at times contentious debate among proponents of biological–biomechanical and psychosocial perspectives. The primary objectives of the symposium were to achieve integration and collaboration as the most promising way to advance research, understanding, prevention, and treatment. During the 3 days, 22 lectures were presented on various aspects of whiplash injury to stimulate discussion, and they were supplemented with short oral presentations from delegates who had submitted abstracts for the symposium.

This book is based on lectures that were presented during the symposium, and all chapters are written by lecturers and their coworkers. Also included here are several chapters written by invited oral presenters from the meeting. We were delighted by the process and the cordial and collegial atmosphere of the meeting. We believe our objectives have been achieved and that the meeting will greatly advance the field. We hope that you will agree and will share our enthusiasm.

Professor Troels S. Jensen and Helge Kasch were gratified with Professor Dennis C. Turk's offer to help in putting the book together. The resulting volume covers the various areas addressed by the speakers and informed by the discussions during the symposium.

In this volume, a multidisciplinary panel of researchers and clinicians who are leading in areas of whiplash injury and pain research present their points of view on subjects ranging from neurobiological mechanisms of pain, clinical pain, and disability assessment to psychosocial aspects, and, furthermore, discuss current and future treatment options for chronic whiplash patients. In particular, this volume provides an overview of current knowledge on:

- Epidemiology
- Clinical aspects of short- and long-term consequences of mild traumatic neck injury

- Background and update for ongoing biomechanical studies in animals, specimens, and humans who sustain neck injuries
- Prospective identification of the risk factors for widespread pain and chronicity after neck injury
- Factors to consider in developing innovative and integrative prevention and intervention programs

Helge Kasch
Dennis C. Turk
Troels S. Jensen

ACKNOWLEDGMENTS

We, as organizers of the Whiplash Research symposium and editors of this volume, would like to gratefully acknowledge the contribution and encouragement of the International Association for the Study of Pain (IASP) in supporting this research symposium. We wish to acknowledge the contributions of each of our colleagues in presenting stimulating lectures, facilitating discussions among the symposium participants, and particularly for their willingness to prepare the chapters that comprise this volume covering the proceedings. Without their collaboration, the success of the meeting and the present text would not have been possible. We would be remiss in not also acknowledging Research Secretary, Helle Obenhausen

Andersen from the Danish Pain Research Center for her outstanding assistance throughout the planning and conduct of the Research Symposium and in the development of this volume.

CONTENTS

CHAPTER 1

Mechanisms of Joint Pain

Hans-Georg Schaible

Pain in the musculoskeletal system is frequent and often chronic. In particular, some diseases of the joint are quite prominent causes of pain, namely, osteoarthitis (OA), rheumatoid arthritis (RA), and gout, and joints are major sites of injuries. In addition, joints may be involved in diseases of the vertebral column, in addition to other structures of the deep tissue.

In joint diseases, pain typically occurs during movements and loading of the joint, thus appearing as mechanical hyperalgesia in the deep tissue. In many cases, mechanical hyperalgesia reflects pathological disturbances of the joint and is thus considered nociceptive. However, some patients also suffer from persistent pain, for example, night pain in advanced OA, and in these cases, a neuropathic component may contribute to the pain (for review see [13]).

In recent years, research into the mechanisms of the clinical features of joint pain has been intensified, and both experimental and clinical studies are now contributing to a better understanding of joint pain. It has become apparent that chronic joint pain is characterized by neuronal processes at all levels of the neural axis (see Fig. 1-1). Furthermore, there is some progress in the exploration of specific pain mechanisms of different joint diseases such as RA and OA. This chapter will focus on the role of cytokines in the generation of joint pain.

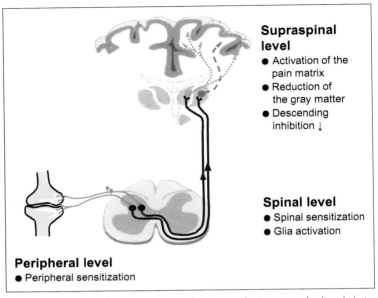

FIGURE 1-1 Overview of neuronal mechanisms that occur during joint diseases.

NEURONAL PROCESSES IN THE NOCICEPTIVE SYSTEM DURING JOINT DISEASE

Fig. 1-1 shows an overview of neuronal mechanisms that occur during joint diseases. At the peripheral level, joint nociceptors are in a sensitized state. The nociceptive sensory fibers show enhanced responses to noxious stimuli and pronounced responses to innocuous stimuli such as movements in the working range and local pressure onto the joint [16]. Peripheral sensitization is a hallmark of all joint diseases. Because some dorsal root ganglion (DRG) neurons show the expression of ATF3 in the monoiodoacetate model of OA, an additional neuropathic pain mechanism was proposed for OA pain [13].

At the spinal level, nociceptive neurons with joint input are often in a state of central sensitization. Sensitized spinal cord neurons exhibit enhanced responses to innocuous and noxious pressure applied to the joint as well as to stimuli applied to adjacent and even remote regions of the leg [16]. The enhanced responsiveness of spinal cord neurons

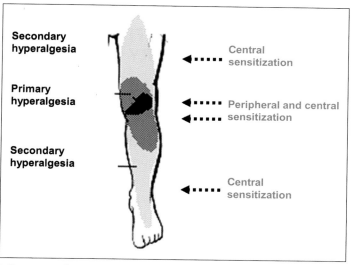

FIGURE 1-2 Areas of primary and secondary hyperalgesia upon inflammation in the knee joint and mechanisms involved.

corresponds to the spreading of pain in patients suffering from RA and OA [1, 3, 11] (see Fig. 1-2). The generation of spinal hyperexcitability results from an increase in the synaptic processing between sensory neurons and spinal cord neurons. In addition, glial cells may be activated and contribute to central sensitization [9].

In the brain, areas involved in the processing of pain are activated. In addition, structural changes were reported. As in other chronic pain states, a reduction of the gray matter was observed in patients suffering from OA. This process is reversible after replacement of the joint. Strikingly, there may be a loss of descending inhibitory activity in the conditioning pain modulation [1, 3, 13]. The reduction of inhibition is thought to contribute to the sensitized state. The loss of conditioning is also reversible after joint replacement [13].

Recent publications on pain in RA patients and OA patients indicate that the contribution of peripheral and central components to the subjective pain experience may vary. For example, the pain may appear preferentially "peripheral" if typical phenomena of central sensitization such as expanded pain areas and temporal summation are weak. Other patients may appear highly "centralized" if such phenomena are strong [1, 3, 11].

PERIPHERAL SENSITIZATION AND PERIPHERAL EFFECTS OF PROINFLAMMATORY CYTOKINES

When primary nociceptive neurons are sensitized, both the channels of transduction and the voltage-gated ion channels, in particular the Na^+ channels, show changes such that the excitability is enhanced [15]. Numerous mediators have the potential to change the responsiveness of sensory neurons, by acting on second messenger systems that change the activation characteristics of ion channels. While earlier research concentrated on mediators such as bradykinin or prostaglandins, more recent research has focused on mediators such as nerve growth factor (NGF) and cytokines. For the role of NGF in the joint, see [2].

It is usually thought that the neutralization of a proinflammatory cytokine attenuates the disease process and as a consequence, the pain is reduced. Careful observation on experimental models and in patients showed, however, that neutralization of a cytokine may reduce the pain quite quickly, well before the attenuation of the disease can be documented [14]. These observations suggest that certain cytokines have a direct role in the generation and maintenance of pain, that is, by targeting the nociceptive system itself. For several proinflammatory cytokines, direct effects on nociceptive neurons were shown: (a) proportions of nociceptive (and other) sensory neurons express receptors for cytokines; (b) in cultured isolated sensory neurons, the application of cytokines may activate second messenger systems, change the excitability, modify ion currents, and regulate molecules involved in nociception; (c) the injection of some cytokines into normal tissue evokes pain behavior in awake animals and enhances the responsiveness of nociceptive sensory fibers; (d) the neutralization of cytokines may reduce pain well in advance of the attenuation of the inflammatory process [14]. Thus, cytokines contribute to pain through an indirect way by the generation of inflammation that causes the release of many mediators acting on neurons, for example, prostaglandins, as well as through a direct way by acting themselves on neurons.

Proinflammatory cytokines such as TNF-α, interleukin-6, interleukin-1β, and interleukin-17 induce a persistent state of sensitization in

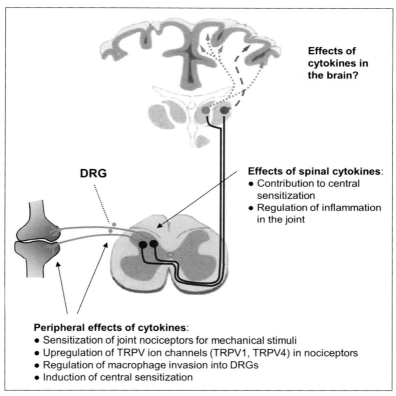

FIGURE 1-3 Effects of cytokines at different neuronal levels.

C fibers of the normal joint (Fig. 1-3). After injection into the normal joint, these cytokines enhance the responsiveness of C fibers to innocuous and noxious movements and local stimulation of the receptive field [14]. However, their effects on Aδ fibers vary. The responses of Aδ fibers of the normal joint are increased by TNF-α, on average unchanged by IL-6 and IL-17, but significantly decreased by IL-1β [14]. Thus, each cytokine has its distinct profile on joint nociceptors. Effects of cytokines may also differ in their reversibility. Effects of TNF-α can be reversed by etanercept. By contrast, sgp130, a molecule that binds to complexes consisting of IL-6 and its soluble receptor (sIL-6R) and thus antagonizes their actions on target cells, prevents the sensitizing effect of IL-6 if applied in a pretreatment protocol, but it does not reverse mechanical hyperexcitability if it is applied once IL-6/sIL-6R complexes have already sensitized the nociceptors [14].

The different effects of cytokines are related to the behavioral consequences of cytokine neutralization in the model of unilateral antigen-induced arthritis (AIA) [14]. Neutralization of TNF significantly reduces mechanical and thermal hyperalgesia within 1–2 days although the inflammatory process is barely reduced after such a short time. Such rapid effects of TNF neutralization were also seen in other inflammatory models and in responsive patients with RA. By contrast, neutralization of IL-6 signaling in the AIA model was mainly effective upon pretreatment and only weakly and late upon posttreatment. Neutralization of IL-17 reduced mechanical hyperalgesia but not thermal hyperalgesia, whereas neutralization of IL-1β only reduced thermal hyperalgesia but not mechanical hyperalgesia. The lack of effect of IL-1β neutralization on mechanical hyperalgesia probably results from the contrasting effects of IL-1β on C- and Aδ- fibers [14]. Fig. 1-4 displays the different pattern of cytokine neutralization in the AIA model.

The different effects of cytokines on mechanical and thermal hyperalgesia raise the question of how these different effects are mediated. First results give a hint that the different effects of cytokines are due to differences in the coupling of intracellular signaling pathways to ion channels of transduction. IL-1β, whose neutralization reduces thermal hyperalgesia, upregulates in DRG neurons in vitro the expression of TRPV1 ion channels, and the anakinra treatment reduces the expression of TRPV1 in DRG neurons in AIA rats [14, 18]. By contrast, IL-17 does not upregulate TRPV1 but increases the expression of TRPV4, an ion channel that exhibits, in addition to thermosensitivity, also some mechanosensitivity and is thought to contribute to mechanical hyperalgesia (for review see [18]).

The direct effect of cytokines on nociceptive nerve fibers has potentially several important consequences. A pain state may reflect not only the disease process in the joint but also the direct impact of

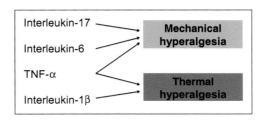

FIGURE 1-4 Different pattern of cytokine neutralization in the AIA model. (From Schaible [14].)

cytokines on the nervous system. Cytokines are also important mediators of neuropathic pain that is originating from injury or disease of neurons themselves [20].

SPINAL SENSITIZATION AND THE ROLE OF PERIPHERAL AND SPINAL PROINFLAMMATORY CYTOKINES IN THIS PROCESS

Spinal cord neurons with input from the knee joint usually have receptive fields in the knee joint (they are activated by mechanical stimuli applied to ligaments and the capsule) and in the lower leg, for example, the ankle. The monitoring of the responses to stimulation of the knee and of the ankle allows one to identify the process of central sensitization. If a spinal neuron shows stronger responses only to the particular input that is enhanced, the increased responses of the spinal cord neuron to this particular stimulus reflect the process of peripheral sensitization. By contrast, if the spinal cord neuron shows enhanced responses to all of its inputs although only one of the inputs is increased, the enhanced responsiveness of the spinal neuron reflects the process of central sensitization. The latter is thought to be the major mechanism underlying secondary hyperalgesia (see Fig. 1-2).

Inflammation of the joint is often associated with peripheral as well as central sensitization (see Fig. 1-2). Key transmitters of spinal sensitization are glutamate and neuropeptides such as substance P. These transmitters are spinally released from sensitized nociceptors. In particular, NMDA receptors for glutamate and neurokinin-1 (NK1) receptors for substance P render postsynaptic neurons hyperexcitable [12, 23]. However, the process of spinal sensitization is modulated by mediators such as prostaglandins and cytokines, which have complex presynaptic and postsynaptic actions. While spinal prostaglandins are produced mainly by neurons [10], cytokines are thought to be produced mainly by glial cells [9].

The injection of TNF-α into the joint cavity of the normal knee joint enhanced the responses of nociceptive spinal cord neurons to stimuli applied to the knee but not to stimuli applied to the ankle. Thus peripheral TNF-α mainly increases the peripheral pain component, but it does not evoke central sensitization, a state in which spinal cord neurons show enhanced responses to stimuli applied to the knee as well as to stimuli applied to the ankle [6]. Notably, the concentration of TNF-α in the joint was significantly increased within the first 4 hours of an acute inflammation in the knee joint evoked by the intra-articular injection of kaolin and carrageenan, thus showing the potential importance of TNF-α in the joint for the responsiveness of spinal cord neurons to mechanical stimulation of the joint [6]. The application of etanercept into the acutely inflamed knee joint significantly reduced the responses of the spinal cord neurons to mechanical stimulation of the inflamed knee, but not the responses to mechanical stimulation of the noninflamed ankle [6]. By contrast, the intra-articular injection of IL-6/sIL6R transienty increased the responses of the neurons to stimuli applied to the knee as well as to the ankle [21]. Thus, the application of IL-6/sIL-6R to the knee joint evoked transiently the whole pattern of central sensitization.

Cytokines also produce effects when they act locally in the spinal cord. Endogenous cytokines may be spinally released from glial cells (and possibly from other cells). The application of either TNF-α [6] or IL-6/sIL-6R [21] to the exposed spinal cord surface enhanced the responses of nociceptive spinal cord neurons with knee input to stimuli applied to the leg, in the absence of knee inflammation. Thus, in addition to prostaglandins, these cytokines enhance the responsiveness of the nociceptive spinal cord neurons to peripheral stimulation. The neutralization of either spinal TNF-α with spinally applied etanercept or an antibody to TNFR1, or of spinal IL-6/sIL-6R with spinally applied sgp130 attenuated the development of spinal sensitization in the model of acute kaolin/carrageenan-induced arthritis. These data show that endogenous spinal TNF-α and IL-6 are involved in the process of spinal sensitization during joint inflammation [6, 21].

Whether the neutralization of the cytokines at the spinal site reverses established hyperexcitability is an intriguing question. Spinal application of etanercept 7–11 hours after induction of kaolin/carrageenan-induced inflammation and spinal sensitization did not significantly reduce the responses of the spinal cord neurons to stimulation of the inflamed joint. In the AIA model, spinal application of etanercept reduced the responses to stimulation of the inflamed joint at day 1 of AIA but not at day 3 of AIA [6]. Neutralization of IL-6/sIL-6R by sgp130 did not reverse spinal cord hyperexcitability [21]. These findings raise the following discussion points. Are the cytokines at the spinal site involved only in the generation of spinal hyperexcitability and not in its maintenance? Do the spinal cytokines induce a state of spinal hyperexcitability that is persistent and not dependent on continuous supply of cytokines? Currently, these questions cannot be answered. Noteworthily, the state of spinal hyperexcitability upon joint inflammation is not totally resistant to reversibility. Selective cyclooxygenase-2 inhibitors can reverse the state of hyperexcitability [19] as well as the spinal application of a specific EP3 receptor agonist [10]. While agonists at the EP2 and the EP4 receptors induce spinal hyperexcitability, the EP3 receptor reduces hyperexcitability once it is established because the EP3 receptor is coupled to pathways counteracting the sensitizing effect [10].

The spinal hyperexcitability is important not only for the generation of pain. Neutralization of spinal TNF-α signaling was shown to reduce the inflammatory process in the joint [22]. This spinal action may be mediated by influencing either dorsal root reflexes (and thus the release of neuropeptides in the joint) or sympathetic reflexes [22]. Whether there are critical time windows for such modulatory effects has not been explored in depth.

FACTORS THAT MAY INFLUENCE THE PERIPHERAL AND CENTRAL PROCESSING OF JOINT NOCICEPTION

Structural Changes of the Innervation of the Joint

It has already been mentioned that chronic pain conditions may be associated with a reduction of the gray matter in brain areas involved in pain processing. Structural changes may also occur in the inflamed joint itself (Fig. 1-5). Based on the analysis of peptidergic fibers, some

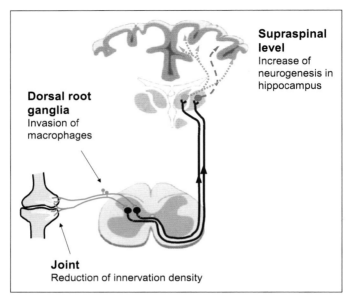

FIGURE 1-5 Factors that may influence the peripheral and central processing of joint nociception.

studies reported a reduction of the density of sensory fibers in the synovial tissue of inflamed joints, whereas others found mainly a loss of sympathetic nerve fibers in arthritic joints, resulting in the prevalence of sensory substance P-positive fibers [17]. In the synovium of human OA joints, a reduction of both sensory and autonomic nerve fibers was found in areas exhibiting synovitis [4]. The reduction of nerve fibers in the superficial synovium was associated with a loss of the dense capillary network that produces the joint effusate [4]. Other authors reported a focal sprouting of nerve fibers at some sites [17]. Whether and how these structural changes contribute to pain generation is unknown. Because nerve fibers express receptive structures along whole fiber branches, a partial reduction of innervation density in the inflamed synovium may not lead to insensitivity of the joints. In the monoiodoacetate model of OA, a neuropathic pain component was reported because a proportion of DRG neurons exhibited an expression of ATF3, and such a neuropathic component could result from nerve fiber damage. It is conceivable, however, that the disturbances of the innervation influence the inflammatory and other pathological processes in the joint. Both sympathetic nerve fibers and sensory nerve fibers act on the tissue and are able to modify the mechanisms of inflammation [17].

Invasion of Macrophages into the DRGs Supplying Inflamed Joints

During inflammation, the joint is heavily infiltrated with immune cells. However, an invasion of macrophages was also observed in the DRGs containing the cell bodies of sensory neurons supplying the inflamed joint [5, 8, 14] (Fig. 1-5). Interestingly, in the unilateral AIA model of the knee, the invasion of the lumbar DRGs was bilateral, that is, on both the inflamed and the noninflamed side. Typically, macrophages invade DRGs and neuronal tissue upon nerve fiber damage, that is, under neuropathic conditions, and macrophages themselves have the potential to destroy neurons. However, in the AIA model, lumbar DRG neurons do not show expression of ATF3, a marker for regeneration after neuronal injury, suggesting that the trigger for invasion was not nerve damage. Rather, it seems to result from an effect of TNF-α because neutralization of TNF-α reduced the invasion of macrophages (Fig. 1-3). In other models, however, some ATF3-expressing DRG neurons were described, namely, in systemic collagen-induced arthritis, the late phase of K/BxN serum transfer arthritis, and the monoiodoacetate model of OA, as already mentioned (for reviews see [8]).

Macrophages achieve different functional states dependent on their activation state. "Classically" activated (M1-) macrophages, typically activated by LPS/interferon-γ, induce inflammation by producing IL-6 and TNF-α, and they can destruct cells by producing NO. By contrast, "alternatively" activated (M2-) macrophages, typically activated by IL-4, produce rather anti-inflammatory cytokines such as IL-10 and are considered important for wound healing. "TNF-α-activated" macrophages are a subtype of M1-macrophages. In AIA, macrophages in the lumbar DRGs were found to exhibit the "TNF-α-activated" phenotype. These macrophages do not express iNOS and do not destroy neurons, but they can activate DRG neurons and causes them to release CGRP [8]. Because in AIA the density of macrophage invasion is correlated with the hyperalgesia, both on the inflamed and on the noninflamed side, the infiltration of lumbar DRGs with macrophages may be involved in the generation of pain. Which role macrophages play in other models of inflammation (dependent on their activation state) should be explored.

Changes of Neurogenesis during Immunization and Arthritis

As alluded to in Fig. 1-1, the gray matter of the brain shows significant changes during arthritis. Neuroplastic changes may also involve alterations of neurogenesis. Throughout life, the adult brain exhibits neurogenesis in the subgranular zone of the mammalian hippocampal dentate gyrus (DG), and neural stem/progenitor cells proliferate into neuronal or glial progenitors. The newly generated neurons migrate into the granule cell layer of the DG and integrate into the existing hippocampal circuitry. They modulate brain performance under altered environmental conditions, and the new cells may contribute to synaptic plasticity and are thought to be involved in long-term potentiation and depression. Adult neurogenesis can be up- or downregulated by a wide variety of factors such as aging, psychosocial and physical stress, irradiation, enriched environment, and physical exercise. Inflammatory conditions, in particular within the central nervous system, inhibit neurogenesis (for review see [7]).

Because inflammation is associated with significantly altered pain and locomotor behavior, we hypothesized that neurogenesis in the DG may be altered. Compared with normal rats, AIA rats showed significantly increased neurogenesis (Fig. 1-5). Interestingly, neurogenesis was similarly enhanced in rats that were only immunized but in which no AIA was induced and that showed normal locomotor behavior and no pain. Thus, enhanced neurogenesis was significantly associated with the immunization process and neither with manifest additional local inflammation alone nor with significant alteration of locomotor behavior and hyperalgesia at the inflamed knee. It may be speculated that enhanced neurogenesis contributes to the generation of disease defense mechanisms. On the other hand, as shown for recovery following stroke, enhanced neurogenesis can also contain elements of maladaptation [7].

CONCLUDING REMARKS

Both the deeper insights into the molecular mechanisms of nociception and the better understanding of the integrative effects of the brain will further our understanding of chronic joint pain. In many aspects, this recent pain research is becoming more disease-related. It is hoped that the multidisciplinary approaches will provide better concepts and better therapeutic approaches to musculoskeletal diseases.

ACKNOWLEDGMENTS

The author thanks the Bundesministerium für Bildung and Forschung (BMBF) and the Deutsche Forschungsgemeinschaft (DFG) for funding the research that is reported in this chapter.

REFERENCES

1. Arendt-Nielsen L, Eskehave TN, Egsgaard LL, Petersen KK, Graven-Nielsen T, Hoeck HC, Simonsen O, Siebuhr AS, Karsdal M, Bay-Jensen AC. Association between experimental pain biomarkers and serologic markers in patients with different degrees of painful knee osteoarthritis. Arthritis Rheum 2014;66:3317–26.

2. Ashraf S, Mapp PI, Burston J, Bennett AJ, Chapman V, Walsh DA. Augmented pain behavioural responses to intra-articular injection of nerve growth factor in two animal models of osteoarthritis. Ann Rheum Dis 2014;73:1710–8.

3. Egsgaard LL, Eskehave TN, Bay-Jensen AC, Hoeck HC, Arendt-Nielsen L. Identifying specific profiles in patients with different degrees of painful knee osteoarthritis based on serological biochemical and mechanistic pain biomarkers: a diagnostic approach based on cluster analysis. Pain 2015;156:96–107.

4. Eitner A, Pester J, Nietzsche S, Hofmann GO, Schaible HG. The innervation of synovium of human osteoarthritic joints in comparison with normal rat and sheep synovium. Osteoarthritis Cartilage 2013;21:1383–91.

5. Inglis J, Nissim A, Lees DM, Hunt SP, Chernajovsky Y, Kidd BL. The differential contribution of tumour necrosis factor to thermal and mechanical hyperalgesia during chronic inflammation. Arthritis Res Ther 2005;7:R807–R816.

6. König C, Zharsky M, Möller C, Schaible HG, Ebersberger A. Involvement of peripheral and spinal tumor necrosis factor α (TNFα) in spinal cord hyperexcitability during knee joint inflammation in rat. Arthritis Rheum 2014;66:599–609.

7. Leuchtweis J, Boettger MK, Niv F, Redecker C, Schaible HG. Enhanced neurogenesis in the hippocampal dentate gyrus during antigen-induced arthritis in adult rat—a crucial role of immunization. PLoS One 2014;9:e89258.

8. Massier J, Eitner A, Segond von Banchet G, Schaible H-G. Effects of differently activated rodent macrophages on sensory neurons: implications for arthritis pain. Arthritis Rheum 2015;67:2263-72. doi: 10.1002/art.39134.

9. McMahon SB, Malcangio M. Current challenges in glia-pain biology. Neuron 2009;64:46–54.

10. Natura G, Bär K-J, Eitner A, Boettger MK, Richter F, Hensellek S, Ebersberger A, Leuchtweis J, Maruyama T, Hofmann GO, et al. Neuronal prostaglandin E2 receptor subtype EP3 mediates antinociception during inflammation. Proceedings Natl Acad Sci USA 2013;110:13648–53.

11. Phillips K, Clauw DJ. Central pain mechanisms in the rheumatic diseases. Arthritis Rheum 2013;65:291–302.

12. Sandkühler J. Learning and memory in pain pathways. Pain 2000;88:113–8.

13. Schaible H-G. Mechanisms of chronic pain in osteoarthritis. Curr Rheumatol Rep 2012;14:549–56.

14. Schaible H-G. Nociceptive neurons detect cytokines in arthritis. Arthritis Res Ther 2014;16:470.

15. Schaible H-G, Ebersberger A, Natura G. Update on peripheral mechanisms of pain: beyond prostaglandins and cytokines. Arthritis Res Ther 2011;13:210.

16. Schaible H-G, Richter F, Ebersberger A, Boettger MK, Vanegas H, Natura G, Vazquez E, Segond von Banchet G. Joint pain. Exp Brain Res 2009;196:153–62.

17. Schaible H-G, Straub RH. Function of the sympathetic supply in acute and chronic experimental joint inflammation. Auton Neurosci 2014;182:55–64.

18. Segond von Banchet G, Boettger MK, König C, Iwakura Y, Bräuer R, Schaible HG. Neuronal IL-17 receptor upregulates TRPV4 but not TRPV1 receptors in DRG neurons and mediates mechanical but not thermal hyperalgesia. Mol Cell Neurosci 2013;52:152–60.

19. Telleria-Diaz A, Schmidt M, Kreusch S, Neubert AK, Schache F, Vazquez E, Vanegas H, Schaible HG, Ebersberger A. Spinal antinociceptive effects of cyclooxygenase inhibition during inflammation: involvement of prostaglandins and endocannabinoids. Pain 2010;148:26–35.

20. Üceyler N, Schäfers M, Sommer C. Mode of action of cytokines on nociceptive neurons. Exp Brain Res 2009;196:67–78.

21. Vazquez E, Kahlenbach J, Segond von Banchet G, König C, Schaible HG, Ebersberger A. Spinal interleukin-6 is an amplifier of arthritic pain. Arthritis Rheum 2012;64:2233–42.

22. Waldburger JM, Firestein GS. Regulation of peripheral inflammation by the central nervous system. Curr Rheumatol Rep 2010;12:370–8.

23. Woolf CJ, Salter MW. Neuronal plasticity: increasing the gain in pain. Science 2000; 288:1765–8.

CHAPTER 2

Pain Signaling Systems from Injured Cervical Facet Joints

Meagan E. Ita and Beth A. Winkelstein

C hronic pain is a common symptom of whiplash-associated injuries. During whiplash, the spine undergoes abnormal motions, and tissue injury of the capsular ligament of the cervical facet joints occurs. Under such pathophysiological loading, peripheral and central neuroimmune and nociceptive signaling cascades are initiated that lead to the onset and maintenance of pain (Fig. 2-1). Pain sensation includes both sensory and emotional experiences, but "nociception" refers to the physiological responses and signal transmission that encodes pain [33]. Typical behavioral signs and symptoms are exhibited by whiplash patients, with allodynia and hyperalgesia to mechanical and thermal stimuli. Allodynia is that pain elicited by a normally non-noxious (nonpainful) stimulus, and hyperalgesia is a heightened response to a noxious (painful) stimulus [33]. These signs are quantifiable and have been used in both clinical studies and animal models of pain, using dermatomal mapping between species. When considering whiplash, the term "injury" is complicated since it may apply to structural injury of tissue in terms of biomechanics, or it may be taken as dysfunction or pain when considering physiological metrics. For the purposes of clarification in this chapter, *injury* encompasses scenarios in which there is pain. Further, the development of facet-mediated

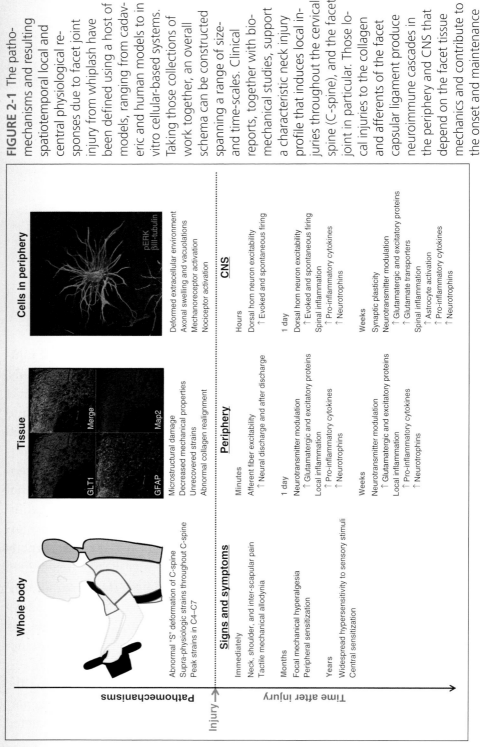

FIGURE 2-1 The pathomechanisms and resulting spatiotemporal local and central physiological responses due to facet joint injury from whiplash have been defined using a host of models, ranging from cadaveric and human models to in vitro cellular-based systems. Taking those collections of work together, an overall schema can be constructed spanning a range of size- and time-scales. Clinical reports, together with biomechanical studies, support a characteristic neck injury profile that induces local injuries throughout the cervical spine (C-spine), and the facet joint in particular. Those local injuries to the collagen and afferents of the facet capsular ligament produce neuroimmune cascades in the periphery and CNS that depend on the facet tissue mechanics and contribute to the onset and maintenance of pain.

Whole body

Abnormal "S" deformation of C-spine
Supra-physiologic strains throughout C-spine
Peak strains in C4–C7

Tissue

Microstructural damage
Decreased mechanical properties
Unrecovered strains
Abnormal collagen realignment

Cells in periphery

pERK
βIII-tubulin

Deformed extracellular environment
Axonal swelling and vacuolations
Mechanoreceptor activation
Nociceptor activation

GLT1 / Merge
GFAP / Map2

Signs and symptoms

Immediately
Neck, shoulder, and inter-scapular pain
Tactile mechanical allodynia

Months
Focal mechanical hyperalgesia
Peripheral sensitization

Years
Widespread hypersensitivity to sensory stimuli
Central sensitization

Periphery

Minutes
Afferent fiber excitability
↑ Neural discharge and after discharge

1 day
Neurotransmitter modulation
↑ Glutamatergic and excitatory proteins
Local inflammation
↑ Pro-inflammatory cytokines
↑ Neurotrophins

Weeks
Neurotransmitter modulation
↑ Glutamatergic and excitatory proteins
Local inflammation
↑ Pro-inflammatory cytokines
↑ Neurotrophins

CNS

Hours
Dorsal horn neuron excitability
↑ Evoked and spontaneous firing

1 day
Dorsal horn neuron excitability
↑ Evoked and spontaneous firing
Spinal inflammation
↑ Pro-inflammatory cytokines
↑ Neurotrophins

Weeks
Synaptic plasticity
Neurotransmitter modulation
↑ Glutamatergic and excitatory proteins
↑ Glutamate transporters
Spinal inflammation
↑ Astrocyte activation
↑ Pro-inflammatory cytokines
↑ Neurotrophins

Pathomechanisms

Time after injury

Injury

whiplash pain symptoms following injury depends on a host of neuroimmune cascades and nociceptive signaling responses, as well as on the magnitude of biomechanical loading of the facet capsule (Fig. 2-1).

This chapter provides an overview of the relationships between biomechanical loading, nociceptive signaling, and pain to describe the relevant physiological responses of the facet joint to mechanical loading in the context of pain, ranging from macroscopic points of view to cellular injuries (Fig. 2-1). It begins with a review of clinical studies summarizing the epidemiology related to cervical facet joint pain from whiplash, and describing those related pain symptoms and the time course of the clinical pain syndrome. Next, biomechanical studies are briefly reviewed, including those of volunteers, full-body cadavers, and cadaveric head–neck preparations; of note, that body of work is quite extensive and far greater than what can be reviewed here [20].

The engineering evidence that implicates the facet joint as having a role in whiplash injury and pain is summarized here. Building off that work, in vivo models are reviewed, particularly those that incorporate biomechanics to understand mechanisms of pain production. In that section, we relate findings regarding pain symptoms with the physiological cascades in both the periphery and the central nervous system (CNS); more exhaustive reviews are provided [6]. Nociceptive signaling can lead to sensitization, which is increased responsiveness of neurons to their normal input or recruitment of a response to normally subthreshold inputs [33]. Sensitization can occur in the periphery or in the CNS. Peripheral sensitization leads to altered nociceptive responses at the injury site, including decreased thresholds for afferent firing and increased responsiveness of peripheral nociceptive neurons; central sensitization involves the increased spontaneous activity and responsiveness of nociceptive neurons in the CNS, which results in increased nociception at *secondary* sites that have no tissue damage [33]. Given the challenges in measuring ligament damage other than gross tissue responses in vivo, we separately present studies that further investigate local mechanotransduction processes by highlighting relationships between locally induced biomechanical deformations and microstructural changes, and the release of pain mediators. Lastly, we conclude this chapter with a brief section highlighting the importance of some of these findings for pain therapies and interventions that specifically target those spatiotemporal neuroimmune cascades that are related to facet-mediated pain. We briefly propose several future directions for research that will further define facet-mediated pain signaling and whiplash mechanisms that can further inform effective clinical diagnostics and treatments.

CLINICAL RELEVANCE

Neck pain is a common and costly medical problem worldwide, and affects around 100 million American adults, with an estimated annual economic cost in the United States of up to $635 billion [18]. Neck pain is the most common symptom reported by patients sustaining whiplash injury, with one-third of whiplash patients reporting symptoms that last for at least 2 years following injury [37]. The cervical facet joints are bilateral joints in the posterolateral region of the spine, and are responsible for coupling rotation and bending in the neck, as well as transmitting axial load [20]. The articulating joint is innervated by the medial branches of the primary dorsal rami of the superior and inferior cervical levels of each joint [3]. Afferent nerve fibers terminate in the facet joint capsule; these include mechanoreceptive and nociceptive C- and Aδ- fibers, with cell bodies in the dorsal root ganglion (DRG) that transmit sensory information from the periphery and terminate in the dorsal horn of the spinal cord [4, 6, 20, 21]. As such, because the facet capsular ligament is rather weak and the facet joint can undergo abnormal motions during whiplash, the facet joints and their capsular ligaments have the potential to generate pain under certain loading conditions.

Patients sustaining whiplash injuries present with pain symptoms and widespread hypersensitivity to mechanical and thermal stimuli that are indicative of CNS sensitization [36, 47, 49]. Pain symptoms from whiplash injury include neck pain and stiffness and have early onset after injury, with many that can persist for at least 2 years [36]. Whiplash patients also exhibit decreased pain thresholds to pressure stimuli over the articular pillars of the cervical spine and in the upper limbs, decreased thermal pain thresholds over the cervical spine, and hypersensitivity during upper limb extension [47, 49]. For example, in a study of 76 whiplash patients, 22.4% of patients reported persistent moderate/severe pain symptoms and demonstrated generalized hypersensitivity to sensory stimuli, which was distinguishable from patients who reported recovered or mild pain [49]. Additionally, while all of those whiplash patients exhibited behavioral sensitivity at 1 month after injury, hyperalgesia persisted at the same severity level for at least 2 years in patients with persistent moderate/severe pain, but it resolved in all of the other patients within 2 months after injury [49]. The existence of localized and focal mechanical hyperalgesia in all whiplash patients early after injury suggests peripheral sensitization of nociceptors, while the generalized hypersensitivity that long outlasts the injury event is likely due to central sensitization.

The facet joints have been implicated as the leading source of pain in patients with chronic whiplash-associated pain in 25–62% of cases via anesthetic nerve blocks or provocative testing [1, 2, 15, 16]. For example, 82 of 128 patients with chronic neck pain who underwent diagnostic blocks to the cervical facets were completely relieved of pain [1]. Pain symptoms are also attenuated by radiofrequency neurotomy, which denervates the cervical facet joints through simulation of the medial branches that innervate them [2]. Provocative testing via joint distension or electrical stimulation of cervical facet joints can also reproduce patient pain in the occiput, neck, and/or shoulders [15, 16], which confirms that mechanical loading of the capsule can activate its nociceptive afferents. These studies reveal the cervical levels most commonly implicated in facet-mediated chronic pain as C2–C3, C5–C6, and C6–C7 [2].

BIOMECHANICAL STUDIES OF VOLUNTEERS, CADAVERS, AND CADAVERIC HEAD–NECK PREPARATIONS

Studies with human volunteers, full-body and/or head–neck cadaveric specimen preparations simulating low-velocity rear-end motor vehicle impacts that are characteristic of the whiplash exposure have collectively defined a signature deformation of the cervical spine. That deformation is initiated within the first 100–120 ms after seat acceleration due to the upward motion of the thorax, which transmits loads to the cervical spine, producing an "S" curvature of the spine [17, 23, 35, 39, 57]. During that whiplash neck kinematic, the lower cervical levels undergo hyperextension and tension anteriorly, while the upper cervical levels undergo flexion [17, 57]. The local intervertebral motions that result from abnormal cervical deformations can induce excessive strains in the cervical facet capsules and other spinal ligaments, with magnitudes that vary across the spinal levels [20]. The strains in the cervical facet capsules are greatest in the lower cervical spine (C4–C7) [9, 17, 40, 41, 50], with the linear strains across the C6/C7 facet joint peaking at 29–40% during accelerations that simulate moderate-to-severe whiplash-associated motor vehicle impacts [41]. Further, for a comparable injury exposure, the lower cervical facets slide anterior–posteriorly parallel to the line of the joint articulation, reaching a maximum relative displacement of 6.0 mm (~51% facet capsular strain as inferred from bony landmarks) [9]. In cadaveric simulations of head restraint contact during rear impacts, the C4/C5 and C5/C6 facets undergo the greatest combined anterior–posterior, superior–inferior displacements of 2.5 ± 1.8 and 2.5 ± 2.3 mm, respectively [50]. Similar translations measured between upper and lower bony facet landmarks have been reported for studies of cadaveric head–neck preparations, with C4/C5 and C6/C7 experiencing the greatest anterior–posterior (5.4 mm) and superior–inferior (2.6 mm) displacements, respectively [41].

Despite being of greater magnitude than those experienced during physiological neck motions, whiplash-induced strains in the cervical facet capsules are not sufficient to induce capsule rupture [40, 41, 56]. In addition, the intervertebral rotations at C6/C7 and C7/T1 during simulated whiplash exceed the physiological limits of rotation [17], with ligament laxity occurring throughout the cervical spine [19] but no evidence of capsule rupture [17, 40, 41, 48, 56]. Interestingly, facet capsule rupture itself, despite being more severe biomechanically, does not induce pain [55]. Taken together with the fact that the facet capsule is richly innervated with mechanosensitive afferents [3, 4, 21], the absence of pain after joint rupture implies that such joint afferents must be intact at injury for facet-mediated pain to develop from facet joint trauma.

During whiplash, capsular deformations are not uniform throughout the cervical spine or regionally on the surface of the capsular ligament. For example, deformations are greatest in the posterior portion of the capsule relative to the anterior portion [50]. Capsular strains are also nonuniform during cervical spine bending, although the principal strains are typically directed along the joint line [54]. Nonuniform strains in the facet capsule have important implications for the mechanosensitive afferents that terminate in that capsule since higher magnitude strains may preferentially activate or injure fibers in specific regions. If these higher magnitude strains load the facet capsule while it remains intact, and thus do not rupture the afferents themselves, a biomechanical environment is created by that *subfailure* loading condition that has the capacity to generate pain.

PHYSIOLOGICAL RELEVANCE OF FACET LOADING AND PAIN SIGNALING

In vivo models using facet capsule stretch comparable to whiplash exposures exhibit persistent behavioral hypersensitivity that mimics the pain symptoms that are observed clinically [29, 31]. These behavioral hypersensitivity signs of pain include mechanical allodynia in the shoulder, neck, and even radiating to the hand (or paw in rodents) that is evident within 1 day after facet joint loading and persists for up to 6 weeks [29, 31]. Further, the magnitude of facet joint stretch (i.e., the severity of the ligament injury) affects the development and extent of pain, with stretches comparable to those sustained during whiplash producing up to a three-fold increase in mechanical allodynia compared with stretches simulating nonpainful physiological motions of the joint [14, 31]. Interestingly, this modulation of injury severity correlating with pain symptoms only holds for subfailure regimes. In other words, for joint loading that produces ligament rupture (failure), pain symptoms are only transient [29, 55]. These findings are consistent with cadaveric whiplash simulations reporting no evidence of capsule rupture [17, 40, 41, 56] and support the hypothesis that subfailure bio-mechanical loading of intact facet capsules can activate afferents and contribute to subsequent pain development.

The afferent fibers that innervate the facet joint and its capsular ligament are activated during, and after, any stretch across the facet joint, at those same magnitudes of biomechanical strain that produce behavioral hypersensitivity [4, 29, 31, 34]. Both low-threshold and high-threshold mechanoreceptors have been demonstrated in the facet capsule of the goat, and their activation and physiological responses have been related to biomechanical metrics like the applied tissue strain [4, 34]; low-threshold mechanoreceptors are activated at physiological strains of 10–15% and high-threshold mechanorecep-tors at significantly greater strains of 25–47%. Furthermore, persistent after-discharge occurs for up to 4 minutes following strains of 38 ± 12% and for longer times following strains of 45 ± 15% [4, 34]. Such stretch of the facet capsule is also associated with altered axon morphology in afferents of the ligament, with axonal swelling and vacuolations [22]. Interestingly, high-threshold mechanoreceptors are activated by strains comparable to those sustained by the cervical facet capsules in the lower cervical spine during whiplash simulations and those sub-catastrophic strains defined in studies of elongation-to-failure using isolated motion segments [4, 48, 54]. The same strain magnitudes that activate these mechanoreceptors are also associated with pain in vivo [29, 31]. Further, silencing the afferent activity local to the joint using the fast-acting anesthetic bupivacaine attenuates pain when given intra-articularly early (4 hours) after painful injury, but not when given at 8 hours or 1 day [5]. These studies suggest that interrupting afferent activity early after joint injury may prevent excitatory signaling that contributes to pain, but that such increases in neuronal excitability that are established within 4–8 hours following injury quickly contribute to central sensitization and pain. This finding has implications for clinical treatment in that it implies that while there may be an interventional window for effective treatment after injury, that time period is quite narrow and may not be pragmatic in clinical practice.

Painful facet capsule injury also induces electrophysiological changes in the dorsal horn of the spinal cord that contributes to an increase in excitatory signaling, modulation of glutamatergic signaling, excitatory synaptogenesis, and the development of central sensitization [5,7,10,42]. Dorsal horn neuronal hyperexcitability and increased spontaneous firing both develop between 6 hours and 1 day following painful facet injury and parallel the development of behavioral hyperalgesia [7, 42]. A functional shift of dorsal horn neurons from low-threshold mechanoreceptors, or nociceptive-specific neurons, to wide dynamic range neurons is also evident after painful facet injury [42]. This phenotypic shift is important since wide dynamic range neurons are activated by a large range of stimuli and can increase amplification of painful stimuli, leading to decreased pain thresholds and behavioral hypersensitivity. Intrathecal gabapentin, which is hypothesized to prevent extracellular calcium influx by acting on the α2δ-1 subunit of voltage-dependent calcium channels, reduces the frequency of evoked neuronal firing in the dorsal horn and attenuates mechanical hyperalgesia in rats following painful facet injury [10]. Because gabapentin reduces overall neuronal activity and it is effective as a therapeutic to attenuate mechanical hyperalgesia, dorsal horn excitability is further implicated in the development of pain.

The glutamatergic system is the primary excitatory signaling system in the nervous system. Modifications throughout that regulatory system, in both the spinal cord and the DRG, increase spontaneous activation of neurons and contribute to central sensitization after painful facet injury [5, 8, 12, 14, 32, 38, 51]. For example, spinal glutamatergic and excitatory proteins, including the ionotropic glutamate receptor N-methyl-D-aspartate (NMDA) subunit (pNR1), the metabotropic glutamate receptor-5 (mGluR5), and the glutamate-aspartate transporter (GLAST), are all upregulated in the spinal cord at the level of painful facet injury; in contrast, the spinal glutamate transporters, excitatory amino acid carrier 1 (EAAC1) and the glutamate transporter 1 (GLT1), primarily localized to astrocytes, are downregulated [5, 12, 14, 51]. This simultaneous increase in glutamatergic excitatory proteins and decrease in glutamate transporters likely contribute to the increase in dorsal horn neuron excitability that is evident after painful facet injury. It further suggests that this excitability may at least partly be due to decreased clearance of glutamate from spinal cord synapses.

Increased excitability in the superficial dorsal horn can also be due to excitatory synaptogenesis, which is an increase in the density of excitatory synapses [8]. Together with early and sustained tactile allodynia, central sensitization is implicated as contributing to pain maintenance.

Nociceptive signaling is also altered in the DRG and spinal cord, with temporal variability and responses dependent on the *magnitude* of mechanical loading to the facet joint [12, 32]. For example, mRNA for the nociceptive neurotransmitter, substance P, increases temporally in the DRG following *nonpainful* injury, but does not change following *painful* injury [32], suggesting that painful injury may induce axonal dysfunction that disrupts protein transport. Expression of the glutamate receptor mGluR5 and its second messenger, protein kinase C-ε (PKCε), also increase in the DRG depending on the magnitude of facet joint tension. Neuronal mGluR5 and PKCε are significantly elevated in the DRG at 1 week after a painful facet injury, but not at an earlier time point [12, 51]. Both PKCε and mGluR5 increase nociceptive afferent excitability in inflammatory pain and are integral components of the nociceptive intracellular signaling cascades. Furthermore, delayed elevation of mGluR5 and PKCε in the DRG suggests that these proteins may play a role in the maintenance, but not the initiation, of pain. EAAC1 expression in the spinal cord is also regulated differentially by the magnitude of facet joint loading; in particular, spinal EAAC1 increases 1 week after nonpainful injury [12], which is contrary to the *decrease* in EAAC1 following painful facet injury [5]. This suggests that tissue injury facilitates spinal plasticity at times when pain is sustained after tissue injury, specifically in association with glutamate receptors and transporters, and thus that the *magnitude* of tissue loading modulates not only pain behavior but also glutamatergic plasticity.

Facet capsule injury directly and indirectly initiates local (peripheral) and central inflammatory cascades through modulation of both glial cells and neurotrophins. Characterization of inflammatory responses following painful facet injury indicates a significant inflammatory response in the spinal cord and DRG from 1 day to 2 weeks following injury [24, 25, 28]. Specifically, expression of glial fibrillary acidic protein (GFAP), an indicator of activated astrocytes, is increased in the spinal cord for at least 2 weeks, although the microglia response is not significantly activated [5, 13, 28]. Proinflammatory cytokines and neurotrophins, such as nerve growth factor (NGF) and brain-derived neurotrophic factor (BDNF), are also involved in signaling and inflammatory cascades, and their expression following painful facet injury parallels pain symptoms [26, 29, 53]. BDNF protein expression increases in the spinal cord and DRG 1 week after facet injury [26]; when a BDNF sequestering molecule, trkB-Fc, is intrathecally injected 5 days after painful loading, however, behavioral sensitivity is partially attenuated within 1 day of treatment [26]. That intrathecal trkB-Fc treatment also decreases phosphorylated ERK (pERK) [26], a secondary signaling molecule and indicator of neuronal activation, which is otherwise increased at that time after painful facet injury [5]. Similar to BDNF, NGF increases after painful facet injury within 1 day of injury in the DRG *and* in the tissues of the joint [53]. In addition, intra-articular injections of NGF alone also induce pain in the absence of any mechanical joint loading [53], which can induce the release of substance P into the dorsal horn. Inhibiting intra-articular NGF signaling via anti-NGF antibody also prevents pain *and* spinal hyperexcitability after painful loading [53]. As such, since modulating both spinal BDNF and intra-articular NGF attenuates pain symptoms, these neurotrophins are further implicated in traumatic facet-mediated pain. Although there is mounting evidence from a variety of experimental and modeling approaches that peripheral biomechanics drive the pain response in facet-mediated trauma-induced pain [6, 20], the specific mechanisms by which injury signals encode that signal to produce chronic pain and/or how they are different from nociceptive pain or mechanosensation are only recently being investigated.

INSIGHTS ABOUT MECHANOTRANSDUCTION OF PAIN IN THE PERIPHERY

The peripheral tissue strains required for pain production in vivo vary substantially with inhomogeneities in the local strain fields. Those same conditions induce microstructural damage in the facet capsular ligament that varies regionally and may drive the pain signaling that leads to facet-mediated loading-induced chronic pain [44]. For example, maximum principal strains in the rat facet capsule range from ~50% in the posterior region to ~35% in the posterolateral region, and ~45% in the lateral region of the capsular ligament [44]. The realignment of collagen fibers in the ligament also shows regional variability; ligament distraction simulating painful facet injury causes significantly greater collagen fiber dispersion in the posterior region than in the lateral region of the capsule [44]. Furthermore, local strains in the capsule do not recover after joint retractions that simulate whiplash, which implies there is permanent microstructural damage [27, 46]. Thresholds for tissue strain to produce pain likely depend on those strain magnitudes that are also associated with microstructural damage in the ligament [43, 45]. In fact, the strains associated with ligament damage (i.e., collagen realignment), correspond to those strains that also produce pain [30], suggesting altered local structural responses may be sufficient to elicit sustained nociceptor firing and ultimately pain. Indeed, substantial inhomogeneous local strain fields induce collagen realignment indicative of microstructural damage in cadaveric specimens, at ligament stretches that are experienced during whiplash [27, 46]. The *local* biomechanical environment of the afferents and neurons innervating the facet capsular ligament modulates their release of pain mediators. In fact, using model systems to apply stretch to neuron-seeded collagen gels, we have begun to simultaneously measure both collagen fiber kinematics and neuron activity in response to macroscopic loading in order to define mechanotransduction of such a local system important in facet-mediated pain. Using that system, we have found that macroscopic stretch simulating painful capsular loading induces collagen realignment and neuronal expression and release of pERK, a secondary signaling molecule and indicator of neuronal activation, both of which exceed those responses after physiological loading (Fig. 2-2) [58]. In fact, neuronal pERK expression is weakly, but significantly, correlated to the strain experienced by the neurons. These data demonstrate that cellular-level pain signaling is initiated by changes in the local biomechanical environment and support the hypothesis that peripheral biomechanics drive the pain signaling response in facet-mediated pain.

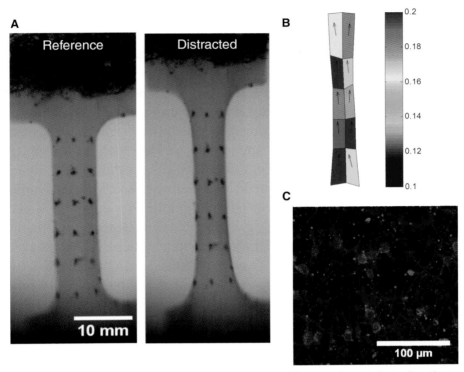

FIGURE 2-2 Neuron–collagen gel constructs enable experimental studies that integrate biomechanics with neuronal and collagen assays to understand the relationship(s) between macroscopic tissue-level and local strains and physiological cellular responses. **A:** Representative images of a neuron–collagen gel showing regional elements in an unloaded (reference) state and following an 8-mm distraction simulating a painful facet injury in vivo (distracted). **B:** The peak strains during loading are measured using optical tracking methods and mapped to the corresponding regional elements. The painful distraction induces strains that vary regionally in the gel and exceed the strain magnitude at which collagen realignment rapidly changes. **C:** A representative image showing an element of the collagen gel after a painful 8 mm distraction, immunolabeled for neurons (*blue*; βIII-tubulin), pERK (*red*), and their colocalization (*pink*), indicating pERK expressed by neurons.

OPPORTUNITIES FOR PAIN INTERVENTION AND FUTURE DIRECTIONS

Those neuronal responses that result from changes in their local biomechanical environment can be blocked or inhibited to prevent the development of pain, offering possibilities for clinical intervention and treatment for whiplash pain. For example, loading-induced pain symptoms in the rat can be attenuated when neuronal activity [5, 7, 10], inflammatory [11, 13], or nociceptive signaling cascades [26, 52, 53] are blocked and/or inhibited. Of course, as briefly reviewed in the previous sections, those cascades develop and progress over different time courses and are modulated by the different factors of the painful facet joint injury. As such, the timing of any therapeutic intervention(s) is critical for successful attenuation and/or abolishment of facet-mediated whiplash pain. For example, silencing afferent activity in the facet joint using the anesthetic bupivacaine attenuates pain symptoms *only* when that treatment is given *before* the development of central sensitization [5]. This finding implies that early neuronal activity in the joint afferents is *required* for the development of persistent pain. Similarly, blocking NGF in the facet using an antibody prevents pain if it is administered *immediately* after the injury [53], but not when administration is delayed for even 1 day, when pain and spinal excitability have already developed. Early NGF activity and signaling in the facet are likely also a requisite for pain development. Taken together, these two examples highlight the involvement of two coordinated but singular mechanisms that offer potential opportunities for targeting. Careful consideration of how these and other initiating events modulate the more complicated and integrated neuroimmune cascades involved in pain in the human is critical in identifying and developing effective therapies with a high clinical translational potential.

As the complicated local and central pain signaling mechanisms become more further elucidated, a clearer picture of the relationship(s) between pain, trauma conditions, and anatomic site for modulation will emerge. While physiological responses to tissue injury are evident locally in the facet, peripherally in the DRG, centrally in the spinal cord, and supraspinally in the brain, pain signaling is first *initiated* by the injurious loading of the afferents that innervate the facet, or by their continued loading due to ligamentous laxity following whiplash. As such, inhibition of those local cascades could prevent peripheral, central, and supraspinal responses observed in facet-mediated pain. Indeed, local mechanotransduction processes involving facet capsular afferents have been suggested as initiating mechanisms of pain, and further defining the relationships between local cell mechanics, physiology, and macroscale strains in the capsular ligament will aid in determining effective local pain interventions. Expanding the knowledge of the macro- and microscale pathomechanisms of facet-mediated trauma-induced pain that contribute to the physiological cascades underlying pain, especially that pain signaling initiated in the facet joint, will provide insight to prevent facet joint injury and treat chronic whiplash pain.

ACKNOWLEDGMENTS

The authors thank Sijia Zhang for providing several panel images. This work was supported by funding from the National Institute of Arthritis, Musculoskeletal and Skin Diseases (#AR056288), the National Institute of Biomedical Imaging and Bioengineering (#EB016638), the Department of Defense (W81XWH-10-2-0140), as well as the Catherine D. Sharpe Foundation.

REFERENCES

1. Aprill C, Bogduk N. The prevalence of cervical zygapophyseal joint pain: a first approximation. Spine (Phila Pa 1976) 1992;17:744–7.

2. Bogduk N. On cervical zygapophysial joint pain after whiplash. Spine (Phila Pa 1976) 2011;36(25, Suppl):S194– S199.

3. Bogduk N, Marsland A. The cervical zygapophysial joints as a source of neck pain. Spine (Phila Pa 1976) 1988;13:610–7.

4. Chen C, Lu Y, Kallakuri S, Patwardhan A, Cavanaugh JM. Distribution of A-δ and C-fiber receptors in the cervical facet joint capsule. J Bone Joint Surg Am 2006;88:1807–16.

5. Crosby ND, Gilliland TM, Winkelstein BA. Early afferent activity from the facet joint after painful trauma to its capsule potentiates neuronal excitability and glutamate signaling in the spinal cord. Pain 2014;155:1878–87.

6. Crosby ND, Smith JR, Winkelstein BA. Pain biomechanics. In: Yoganandan N, Nahum AM, Melvin JW, editors. Accidental injury. New York, NY: Springer-Verlag; 2015. pp. 549–80.

7. Crosby ND, Weisshaar CL, Winkelstein BA. Spinal neuronal plasticity is evident within 1 day after a painful cervical facet joint injury. Neurosci Lett 2013;542:102–6.

8. Crosby ND, Zaucke F, Kras JV, Dong L, Luo ZD, Winkelstein BA. Thrombospondin-4 and excitatory synaptogenesis promote spinal sensitization after painful mechanical joint injury. Exp Neurol 2015;264:111–20.

9. Deng B, Begeman PC, Yang KH, Tashman S, King AI. Kinematics of human cadaver cervical spine during low speed rear-end impacts. Stapp Car Crash J 2000;44: 171–88.

10. Dong L, Crosby ND, Winkelstein BA. Gabapentin alleviates facet-mediated pain in the rat through reduced neuronal hyperexcitability and astrocytic activation in the spinal cord. J Pain 2013;14:1564–72.

11. Dong L, Guarino BB, Jordan-Sciutto KL, Winkelstein BA. Activating transcription factor 4, a mediator of the integrated stress response, is increased in the dorsal root ganglia following painful facet joint distraction. Neuroscience 2011;193:377–86.

12. Dong L, Quindlen JC, Lipschutz DE, Winkelstein BA. Whiplash-like facet joint loading initiates glutamatergic responses in the DRG and spinal cord associated with behavioral hypersensitivity. Brain Res 2012;1461:51–63.

13. Dong L, Smith JR, Winkelstein BA. Ketorolac reduces spinal astrocytic activation and PAR1 expression associated with attenuation of pain after facet joint injury. J Neurotrauma 2013;30:818–25.

14. Dong L, Winkelstein BA. Simulated whiplash modulates expression of the glutamatergic system in the spinal cord suggesting spinal plasticity is associated with painful dynamic cervical facet loading. J Neurotrauma 2010;174:163–74.

15. Dwyer A, Aprill C, Bogduk N. Cervical zygapophyseal joint pain patterns. I: a study in normal volunteers. Spine (Phila Pa 1976) 1990;15:453–7.

16. Fukui S, Ohseto K, Shiotani M, Ohno K, Karasawa H, Naganuma Y, Yuda Y. Referred pain distribution of the cervical zygapophyseal joints and cervical dorsal rami. Pain 1996;68:79–83.

17. Grauer JN, Panjabi MM, Cholewicki J, Nibu K, Dvorak J. Whiplash produces an S-shaped curvature of the neck with hyperextension at lower levels. Spine (Phila Pa 1976) 1997;22:2489–94.

18. Institute of Medicine of the National Academies. Relieving pain in America. Washington, DC: National Academies Press; 2011.

19. Ivancic PC, Ito S, Tominaga Y, Rubin W, Coe MP, Ndu AB, Carlson EJ, Panjabi MM. Whiplash causes increased laxity of cervical capsular ligament. Clin Biomech 2008;23:159–65.

20. Jaumard NV, Welch WC, Winkelstein BA. Spinal facet joint biomechanics and mechanotransduction in normal, injury and degenerative conditions. J Biomech Eng 2011;133:071010.

21. Kallakuri S, Singh A, Chen C, Cavanaugh JM. Demonstration of substance P, calcitonin gene-related peptide, and protein gene product 9.5 containing nerve fibers in human cervical facet joint capsules. Spine (Phila Pa 1976) 2004;29:1182–6.

22. Kallakuri S, Singh A, Lu Y, Chen C, Patwardhan A, Cavanaugh JM. Tensile stretching of cervical facet joint capsule and related axonal changes. Eur Spine J 2008;17:556–63.

23. Kaneoka K, Ono K, Inami S, Hayashi K. Motion analysis of cervical vertebrae during whiplash loading. Spine (Phila Pa 1976) 1999;24:763–70.

24. Kras JV, Dong L, Winkelstein BA. The prostaglandin E2 receptor, EP2, is upregulated in the dorsal root ganglion after painful cervical facet joint injury in the rat. Spine (Phila Pa 1976) 2013;38:217–22.

25. Kras JV, Dong L, Winkelstein BA. Increased interleukin-1α and prostaglandin E_2 expression in the spinal cord at 1 day after painful facet joint injury: evidence of early spinal inflammation. Spine (Phila Pa 1976) 2014;39:207–12.

26. Kras JV, Weisshaar CL, Quindlen J, Winkelstein BA. Brain-derived neurotrophic factor is upregulated in the cervical dorsal root ganglia and spinal cord and contributes to the maintenance of pain from facet joint injury in the rat. J Neurosci Res 2013;91:1312–21.

27. Lee DJ, Winkelstein BA. The failure response of the human cervical facet capsular ligament during facet joint retraction. J Biomech 2012;45:2325–9.

28. Lee KE, Davis MB, Mejilla RM, Winkelstein BA. In vivo cervical facet capsule distraction: mechanical implications for whiplash & neck pain. Stapp Car Crash J 2004;48:1–23.

29. Lee KE, Davis MB, Winkelstein BA. Capsular ligament involvement in the development of mechanical hyperalgesia after facet joint loading: behavioral and inflammatory outcomes in a rodent model of pain. J Neurotrauma 2008;25:1383–93.

30. Lee KE, Franklin AN, Davis MB, Winkelstein BA. Tensile cervical facet capsule ligament mechanics: failure and subfailure responses in the rat. J Biomech 2006;39:1256–64.

31. Lee KE, Thinnes JH, Gokhin DS, Winkelstein BA. A novel rodent neck pain model of facet-mediated behavioral hypersensitivity: implications for persistent pain and whiplash injury. J Neurosci Methods 2004;137:151–9.

32. Lee KE, Winkelstein BA. Joint distraction magnitude is associated with different behavioral outcomes and substance P levels for cervical facet joint loading in the rat. J Pain 2009;10:436–45.

33. Loeser JD, Treede RD. The Kyoto protocol of IASP basic pain terminology. Pain 2008;137:473–7.

34. Lu Y, Chen C, Kallakuri S, Patwardhan A, Cavanaugh JM. Neural response of cervical facet joint capsule to stretch: a study of whiplash pain mechanism. Stapp Car Crash J 2005;49:49–65.

35. Luan F, Yang KH, Deng B, Begeman PC, Tashman S, King AI. Qualitative analysis of neck kinematics during low-speed rear-end impact. Clin Biomech 2000;15:649–57.

36. Maimaris C, Barnes MR, Allen MJ. "Whiplash injuries" of the neck: a retrospective study. Injury 1988;19:393–6.

37. Manchikanti L, Boswell MV, Singh V, Pampati V, Damron KS, Beyer CD. Prevalence of facet joint pain in chronic spinal pain of cervical, thoracic, and lumbar regions. BMC Musculoskelet Disord 2004;5:15.

38. Ohtori S, Takahashi K, Moriya H. Calcitonin gene-related peptide immunoreactive DRG neurons innervating the cervical facet joints show phenotypic switch in cervical facet injury in rats. Eur Spine J 2003;12:211–5.

39. Ono K, Kaneoka K, Wittek A, Kajzer J. Cervical injury mechanism based on the analysis of human cervical vertebral motion and head-neck-torso kinematics during low speed rear impacts. Stapp Car Crash J 1997;41:339–56.

40. Panjabi MM, Cholewicki J, Nibu K, Grauer J, Vahldiek M. Capsular ligament stretches during in vitro whiplash simulations. J Spinal Disord Tech 1998;11:227–32.

41. Pearson AM, Ivancic PC, Ito S, Panjabi MM. Facet joint kinematics and injury mechanisms during simulated whiplash. Spine (Phila Pa 1976) 2004;29:390–7.

42. Quinn KP, Dong L, Golder FJ, Winkelstein BA. Neuronal hyperexcitability in the dorsal horn after painful facet joint injury. Pain 2010;151:414–21.

43. Quinn KP, Lee KE, Ahaghotu CC, Winkelstein BA. Structural changes in the cervical facet capsular ligament: potential contributions to pain following subfailure loading. Stapp Car Crash J 2007;51:1–19.

44. Quinn KP, Winkelstein BA. Cervical facet capsular ligament yield defines the threshold for injury and persistent joint-mediated neck pain. J Biomech 2007;40:2299–306.

45. Quinn KP, Winkelstein BA. Altered collagen fiber kinematics define the onset of localized ligament damage during loading. J Appl Physiol 2008;105:1881–8.

46. Quinn KP, Winkelstein BA. Detection of altered collagen fiber alignment in the cervical facet capsule after whiplash-like joint retraction. Ann Biomed Eng 2011;39:2163–73.

47. Scott D, Jull G, Sterling M. Widespread sensory hypersensitivity is a feature of chronic whiplash-associated disorder but not chronic idiopathic neck pain. Clin J Pain 2005;21:175–81.

48. Siegmund GP, Myers BS, Davis MB, Bohnet HF, Winkelstein BA. Human cervical motion segment flexibility and facet capsular ligament strain under combined posterior shear, extension and axial compression. Stapp Car Crash J 2000;44:159–70.

49. Sterling M, Jull G, Vicenzino B, Kenardy J. Sensory hypersensitivity occurs soon after whiplash injury and is associated with poor recovery. Pain 2003;104:509–17.

50. Sundararajan S, Prasad P, Demetropoulos CK, Tashman S, Begeman PC, Yang KH, King AI. Effect of head-neck position on cervical facet stretch of post mortem human subjects during low speed rear end impacts. Stapp Car Crash J 2004;48:331–72.

51. Weisshaar CL, Dong L, Bowman AS, Perez FM, Guarino BB, Sweitzer SM, Winkelstein BA. Metabotropic glutamate receptor-5 and protein kinase C-epsilon increase in dorsal root ganglion neurons and spinal glial activation in an adolescent rat model of painful neck injury. J Neurotrauma 2010;27:2261–71.

52. Weisshaar CL, Winkelstein BA. Ablating spinal NK1-bearing neurons eliminates the development of pain and reduces spinal neuronal hyperexcitability and inflammation from mechanical joint injury in the rat. J Pain 2014;15:378–86.

53. Winkelstein BA, Kras JV. Intra-articular nerve growth factor initiates pain and associated spinal neuronal hyperexcitability from cervical joint pain. Cervical Spine Research Society Annual Meeting, Paper #17. Orlando, FL; December 2014.

54. Winkelstein BA, Nightingale RW, Richardson WJ, Myers BS. The cervical facet capsule and its role in whiplash injury: a biomechanical investigation. Spine (Phila Pa 1976) 2000;25:1238–46.

55. Winkelstein BA, Santos DG. An intact facet capsular ligament modulates behavioral sensitivity and spinal glial activation produced by cervical facet joint tension. Spine (Phila Pa 1976) 2008;33:856–62.

56. Yoganandan N, Pintar FA. Inertial loading of the human cervical spine. J Biomech Eng 1997;119:237–40.

57. Yoganandan N, Pintar FA, Cusick JF. Biomechanical analyses of whiplash injuries using an experimental model. Accid Anal Prev 2002;34:663–71.

58. Zhang S, Barocas VH, Winkelstein BA. Local neuronal loading modulates pERK expression in a neuron-collagen gel construct simulating facet capsule injury. 7th World Congress of Biomechanics, #W229. Boston, MA; July 2014.

CHAPTER 3

Morphology and Whiplash Injuries

Brian D. Stemper and Brian D. Corner

Whiplash injuries lead to significant worldwide disability, affecting a variety of individuals from younger to older age groups, men and women, and vehicle occupants of varying sizes. Across a number of clinical investigations, it has become clear that certain populations report significantly higher numbers of whiplash injuries. This implies an underlying cause for increased susceptibility in those groups. The cause is likely to include biomechanical, anatomical, physiological, psychological, or sociological factors. The most often cited group of individuals with high susceptibility is the female gender. Women have been consistently identified as being more susceptible to whiplash injuries than men. In fact, clinical and epidemiological literature has indicated that women are 1.4–3.0 times more likely to sustain whiplash injury [7, 11, 27, 28, 31, 40]. Experimental research has, for the most part, supported this clinical finding by identifying different biomechanics of the head, neck, and cervical spine in female volunteers and postmortem human subjects (PMHS). Explanations for these biomechanical differences have included differing body anthropometry, spinal kinematics, or cervical spine geometry between men and women. This chapter outlines biomechanical differences between men and women subjected to low velocity rear impacts, and highlights possible biomechanical and morphological explanations.

Literature reviewed is not intended to be comprehensive, but to outline concepts related to biomechanical susceptibility.

BIOMECHANICS OF WHIPLASH INJURIES

A fundamental understanding of head–neck and cervical spine biomechanics during low velocity rear impacts is required to understand the method by which biomechanical differences between men and women affect the risk and severity of injury. Low-speed automobile rear-impact collisions lead to motions of the occupant's head–neck complex that are unique to other vehicular loading vectors (i.e., frontal or side impact). These motions were studied on the occupant, component, and spinal levels using experimental and computational modeling techniques. At the occupant level, the impacted vehicle is accelerated forward, and the seat begins to interact with the occupant primarily through the seat back. The seat back begins to drive the occupant's thorax anteriorly. However, inertia of the body deforms the seat back, and deflects it rearward. Deflection magnitude is dependent upon the mass and sitting height of the occupant, as well as the seat back characteristics. Eventually, the seat back overcomes the inertial loads from the torso and begins to rebound forward, driving the occupant's body forward and eventually into the shoulder harness of the seat belt.

Occupant interactions with the seat back, as described above, drive head–neck biomechanics during the rear impact, which, in turn, produce signature kinematics of the cervical spine. Specifically, torso interaction with the seat back results in anterior acceleration of the thorax [49], which is quantified at the upper thoracic level (i.e., T1) [59, 71]. The magnitude of anterior thoracic acceleration is generally correlated with the rear-impact severity, measured as the forward acceleration or change in velocity (δ-V) of the vehicle. The head lags as the thorax is accelerated anteriorly because there are no forces placed on the head during the initial stages of the impact. This leads to retraction motion of the head relative to the thorax, which is characterized as posterior displacement of the head without an appreciable change in angular orientation (i.e., flexion or extension) [38, 39]. As the magnitude of retraction motion increases, forces are eventually transferred up the cervical spine, and the head begins to rotate posteriorly into extension to strike the head restraint. Smaller head-to-head restraint horizontal distances (i.e., backset) or active head restraint designs can lead to head restraint contact during the retraction phase and prior to head rotation. Rebound from the head restraint occurs and the head rotates forward into flexion. Forward flexion is eventually limited by contraction of the neck muscles or chin-to-chest interaction.

Inertial loading of the head–neck complex drives cervical spine kinematics during the rear impact. Head retraction produces the signature S-shaped curvature of the cervical spine, which is characterized by flexion at cranial cervical segments (i.e., C0–C3) and extension at caudal segments (i.e., C3–C7), with a transition region in the middle cervical spine (Fig. 3-1) [23, 53]. This nonphysiologic curvature results in abnormal and increased motions of the facet joints that can produce elevated strains in the capsular ligaments [33, 37, 52, 54] that may exceed subcatastrophic failure thresholds [43] and initiate a nociceptive response [12]. Other cervical spine injury theories center around the retraction phase/S-shaped curvature of the cervical spine or head extension phase, and include localized hyperextension resulting in injury to anterior spinal structures [9, 58, 71], and pressure gradients in the cervical spinal canal that can produce nerve root injury [1, 3, 64].

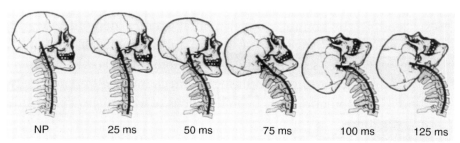

NP   25 ms   50 ms   75 ms   100 ms   125 ms

FIGURE 3-1 The phases of cervical spine kinematics during a low velocity vehicular rear impact include an S-shaped curvature between 25 and 100 ms after the initiation of thoracic acceleration that is characterized by flexion at cranial segments and extension at caudal segments. (Used with permission from Grauer et al. [23].)

The remainder of this chapter will focus on developing an understanding of how occupant and cervical spine morphology can affect rear impact biomechanics, as outlined above. These comparisons will be primarily focused on gender due to the inherent differences in body shape/size between men and women, and the significant amount of research dedicated to that factor.

EVIDENCE OF GREATER SUSCEPTIBILITY

Gender differences provide a suitable model for investigation of morphology-related differences in cervical spine biomechanics during low velocity rear impacts. Although other differences exist, as highlighted below, average female body size is smaller than that of men for a majority of metrics [19, 20]. Outlining metrics specific to rear impact biomechanics is a primary focus of this chapter. However, the case for increased female susceptibility must be made, and an understanding of biomechanical differences between men and women subjected to low velocity rear impact must be provided prior to outlining differences in morphology that can contribute to those changes.

Clinical studies have provided sufficient evidence to indicate that female occupants of motor vehicles sustain a higher number of whiplash injuries. However, due to the focus on injured patients and an inability to control or measure exposure characteristics, those studies provide limited information on the mechanism by which women become more susceptible. In contrast, experimental studies demonstrate specific biomechanical changes between men and women that can contribute to greater injury susceptibility during highly repeatable and identical exposures. Accordingly, outlining biomechanical differences between those two populations has been the focus of a number of experimental investigations.

Experimental investigations that have defined biomechanical differences between men and women have included human volunteers, PMHS, and computational modeling. Studies incorporating volunteers have recreated rear impact accelerations up to 8 km/h using vehicles [4] or horizontal acceleration sleds [6]. Due to ethical considerations, those studies were intentionally focused on producing rear impacts below the threshold for injury. Nonetheless, the clinical condition of the volunteers prior to and following experimentation was reported. Although sample sizes were generally small and statistical analysis was limited, Brault and colleagues [5] identified a significantly longer time period until recovery from initial whiplash-type symptoms (12 compared to 2 hours) following 4 km/h rear impacts. Duration of symptoms was also greater in women following 8 km/h rear impacts (24 compared to 8.8 hours), although not statistically significant.

From a biomechanical standpoint, studies incorporating human volunteers also reported significant differences in head–neck and torso kinematics between men and women. For example, although initial head-to-head restraint distance (i.e., backset) was typically shorter [6, 65], female volunteers demonstrated horizontal head accelerations with higher magnitude and earlier peak values than their male counterparts [6, 24, 31]. Smaller backset was thought to be the result of shorter sitting height in female volunteers, which placed the head closer to the posteriorly inclined head restraint than in men (Fig. 3-2) [6]. Female volunteers also demonstrated greater thoracic acceleration than men [6, 24, 31]. This finding is of particular interest in the light of rear impact severity being identical for male and female volunteers. Greater thoracic accelerations indicate that the driving force for head–neck inertial loading was greater in women when subjected to identical rear impacts than in men. An explanation for this finding was hypothesized to be that women generally had lower body mass and a lower center of mass that contributed to decreased compression of the seat back foam/springs and an overall decrease in seat back deflection due to a shorter moment arm with regard to the pivot point [69]. Therefore, the seat back absorbed less energy, and female occupants experienced more severe loading of the head–neck complex for the same rear impact severity.

Significant differences in cervical spine biomechanics were also identified between men and women. Using a limited number of male and female volunteers and high-speed X-ray imaging, Ono and colleagues [35] identified exaggerated S-shaped curvature in the cervical spines of female volunteers ($n = 2$) compared to their male counterparts ($n = 4$).

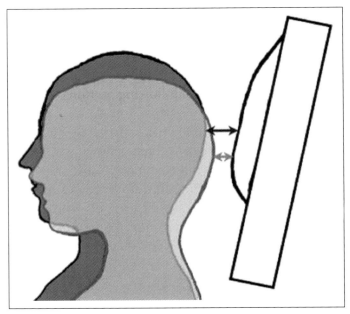

FIGURE 3-2 Studies have identified decreased backset in women due to their relatively shorter sitting height and rearward sloping seat back. However, injury risk remains higher in women than in men. (Used with permission from Carlsson et al. [6].)

Stemper and colleagues [53] incorporated intact head–neck specimens and demonstrated significantly ($P < 0.05$) greater cervical spine intervertebral rotations and enhanced cervical S-curvature. The same group also reported significantly greater absolute facet joint motions [54] and significantly greater facet joint motions normalized by the magnitude of segmental extension [56] in female volunteers. The importance of measuring spinal kinematics lies in the indirect quantification of soft tissue distortion. Intervertebral motions lead to a specific pattern of soft tissue distortion. Extension results in tension of anterior tissues, whereas flexion leads to tension of the posterior tissues. Inertial loading of the head–neck complex during low velocity rear impacts involves a large component of shear force [49], which leads to shear loading across the entire joint that is resisted in large part by the facet joint capsular ligaments due to their sagittal orientation in the cervical spine [36]. Quantification of these motions provides an indirect measure of tissue distortion and injury risk, with greater motions associated with a greater risk or severity of soft tissue injury. Therefore, greater spinal motions demonstrate greater injury risk for women subjected to identical rear impact loading. Possible explanations for those differences are provided in the following sections.

SEATING GEOMETRY AND ANTHROPOMETRY

In 2003, Farmer and colleagues [15] reported that newer head restraint designs with active mechanisms or improved geometric attributes were reducing the risk of whiplash injury among women while having very little effect on male drivers. While clinical studies since that time continue to demonstrate female preponderance [28, 61], changes in women more than in men point to a fundamental difference in automobile seat interaction with the occupant. Seats are designed under a "one size fits all" approach and must provide protection for adult occupants of all sizes from the 5th percentile woman (59-inch stature, 108-pound body weight) to the 95th percentile man (74-inch stature, 223-pound body weight) and beyond. However, automobile safety is often based on the 50th percentile male, meaning that occupants with body sizes further away from that size may not be as well protected.

Given identical seat configurations, experimental studies reported that head-to-head restraint backset in women was less than in men due to rearward incline of automobile seats and decreased sitting height for average women compared to average men. Sitting height for average women is 2.4 inches shorter than sitting height for average men [19, 20]. This means that the posterior aspect of the head for the comparatively shorter woman is positioned closer to the rearward sloping head restraint than the posterior aspect of the male head (Fig. 3-2). Studies demonstrated that decreased backset is associated with decreased injury risk [32, 55, 66]. Therefore, it would be logical to assume that decreased backset in female occupants should be associated with a lower injury risk. However, clinical studies demonstrate that this is not the case.

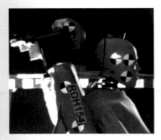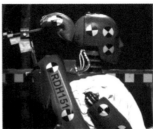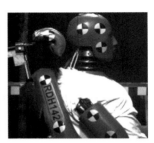

FIGURE 3-3 Vertical mismatch between the sitting height of the occupant and head restraint position may be one explanation for increased injury risk in female occupants. (Used with permission from DeRosia et al. [10].)

A possible explanation for greater injury risk during low velocity rear impacts may be the method by which women interact with the seat back and head restraint. The concept of vertical mismatch in head-to-head restraint positioning was advanced by DeRosia and colleagues [10], and may explain higher injury risk in female occupants that may have smaller backset relative to their taller male counterparts (Fig. 3-3). From a geometric standpoint, if a vertical mismatch exists, the head and neck can be subjected to increased forces or bending moments as the head is either extended over the top of a head restraint that is too low, in the case of a tall occupant, or strikes the seat back and is pushed up into contact with a head restraint that is too high, in the case of a shorter occupant. Either of those cases increases bending moments on the cervical spine, which increases injury risk. Rear impact injury criteria generally included neck bending moments to assess injury risk, with increased bending moments associated with a higher risk [14, 41].

With regard to seating geometry and anthropometry, another possible explanation for greater female susceptibility during rear impacts is related to the location of the body center of mass relative to the seat, as described earlier [69]. This concept is based on the energy-absorbing capacity of the seat back due to rearward deflection about the pivot point during rear impact. As the vehicle is accelerated forward, the occupant's inertia pushes back against the seat back. This leads to compression of the foam/springs and rearward deflection of the seat back. Both of these attributes absorb energy from the impact and decrease the severity of the impact for the occupant. For a given rear impact severity, greater compression of the foam/springs and deflection of the seat back leads to greater energy absorbing effect. Being inertially driven, the magnitude of energy absorption is dependent upon the occupant's torso mass and center of gravity. Greater mass and a center of gravity located further away from the pivot point will contribute to greater energy absorption and a decreased overall severity of the rear impact for the occupant. Average female body mass is 20% lighter than average male body mass, and torso height for an average-sized women is 8% shorter than the after-sized man [19, 20]. Therefore, the ability to deflect the seat back is decreased in women, who experience a more severe rear impact for a given vehicle impact change in velocity.

This section has demonstrated that mismatches between vehicle seat sizes and occupant anthropometry may contribute to a greater injury risk for female occupants. Shorter sitting height can lead to interaction of the head restraint with the occupant's head that can increase flexion moments and contribute to higher injury risk. Likewise, decreased body mass and shorter center of torso mass in women result in decreased seat back deflection and lower energy absorption. While these differences illustrate possible reasons for greater female susceptibility in low velocity rear impacts, they do not explain biomechanical findings outlined in human volunteer testing described above. For example, greater head accelerations are not likely the result of these issues. Therefore, the next section will explore possible head–neck and cervical spine anatomical variations between men and women that may contribute to these differences.

EFFECTS OF ANATOMICAL VARIATIONS

Differences in head–neck and spinal anatomy alter the biomechanical response of the occupant to low velocity rear impacts. Anatomical studies have highlighted gender-based differences that change the head–neck loading pattern, and the method by which the cervical spine responds to inertial loading. Those concepts are highlighted in this section.

Differences in Head and Neck Morphology

Differences in head–neck anthropometry between men and women are often cited as an explanation for greater female susceptibility. Women are thought to have a more slender neck, characterized by an increased length-to-area ratio. Analysis of anthropometric data supports this assertion, in that women have a 2.7% shorter neck length but 16.6% smaller neck circumference [20]. These differences contribute to a more slender female neck that, according to column mechanics, is less capable of carrying loads. Other studies focused on the relationship between head and neck circumference to explain greater female susceptibility, as head mass drives cervical spine inertial loading during rear impacts. In 1972, States and colleagues [46] identified that women have a smaller ratio of head mass to neck cross-sectional area than men, which may explain the increased incidence of whiplash injuries in the female population. That ratio was 31% greater in average women compared to average men [19], with a similarly sized head atop a comparatively smaller neck in women. This leads to more severe head–neck and cervical spine inertial loading during a rear impact and may contribute to greater injury susceptibility in women.

A recently completed large-scale anthropometric survey of U.S. Army soldiers [19] contains additional relevant head and neck anthropometry to elucidate male/female scaling. The 2012 U.S. Army Anthropometric Survey II (ANSUR2) contains 93 standard anthropometric dimensions for 4082 men and 1986 women. Subject ages ranged from 17 to 58 years, with a majority between 20 and 30 years. Head measurements included head circumference, breadth, length, and height (tragion to top of head); and face length and breadth. Neck measurements were neck circumference at infrathyroid and circumference at neck base. Values for neck length were derived from stature, cervicale height, suprasternale height, and head height [67]. Length from tragus to sternal notch (suprasternale) was computed as stature minus sternal notch height minus tragion–top of head height. Similarly, tragus to C7 (cervicale) was computed as stature minus cervicale height minus tragion–top of head height.

Head and neck measurements were significantly different between men and women (Table 3-1). However, large sample sizes may

TABLE 3-1 **Comparison of Male and Female Anthropometry from the U.S. Army ANSUR2 Data set**

	CervHt	HdBr	HdCrc	HdLen	NkCrc	NkCrcBase	Stature	SupraStHt	TrTOH	Wt (kg)	NkLenStrn	NkLenC7
Mal mean	1517.3	154.3	574.4	199.5	397.6	434.6	1756.2	1438.6	131.1	85.5	186.5	107.8
Mal SD	63.3	5.5	16.0	7.0	25.8	25.7	68.6	61.2	6.2	14.2	13.9	12.7
Fem mean	1395.7	147.8	561.1	189.8	329.8	371.2	1628.5	1329.7	126.5	67.8	172.3	106.3
Fem SD	59.5	5.2	19.4	7.4	19.2	19.7	64.2	57.2	6.5	11.0	13.5	11.8
F–M	**–121.6**	**–6.6**	**–13.3**	**–9.7**	**–67.9**	**–63.4**	**–127.7**	**–108.9**	**–4.7**	**–17.8**	**–14.2**	**–1.4**
%F/M	–8.0%	–4.2%	–2.3%	–4.8%	–17.1%	–14.6%	–7.27%	–7.6%	–3.6%	–20.8%	–7.6%	–1.3%
Allow err	7	2	3	2	6	8	6	5	4	0.3	NA	NA
P value	0.0000	0.0000	0.0000	0.0000	0.0000	0.0000	0.0000	0.0000	0.0000	0.0000	0.0000	0.0000
Bonf.01/12	0.0008	0.0008	0.0008	0.0008	0.0008	0.0008	0.0008	0.0008	0.0008	0.0008	0.0008	0.0008

Note: Differences in male and female means are bolded. T-tests of significance and Bonferroni correction are provided. Allowable error established for the ANSUR2 survey is given also. Body weight is in kilograms; otherwise, measurements are in millimeters.

lead to statistical significance for small measurement differences. To confirm that statistically significant differences were relevant, measurement differences were compared with the allowable error established for the study. Measurements were considered relevant if differences were greater than allowable error. In all cases, ANSUR2 male body dimensions were larger than female dimensions. The derived neck length measurements were significantly different between men and women; however, C7 to tragus length (NkLenC7) differed by 1.4 mm, which was less than allowable error when compared to body dimensions of similar magnitude including head height (4 mm) or head length (2 mm).

Vasavada and colleagues [67] provided a plot of male and female head circumference by body weight. The plot clearly showed an upward shift of the male data relative to women. A similar plot of ANSUR2 male and female neck circumference by body weight incorporates log neck circumference by log body weight to better match standard interpretations of allometry (Fig. 3-4).

In a bivariate log–log plot, a y-intercept change without a slope change indicates a difference in overall size without change in proportion [22].

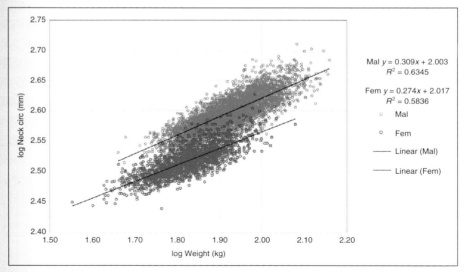

FIGURE 3-4 Log–log plot of male and female neck circumference (mm) by body weight (kg) with regression lines by sex. Relative shift of male and female data indicate a neck circumference size difference. Analysis of covariance confirms a statistical difference in regression line slope.

The plot of male and female log body weight against log neck circumference (Fig. 3-4) displays a shift in intercept and differences in slope. An analysis of covariance confirmed a statistically significant slope difference [45], which indicated a departure from geometric scaling of neck circumference between men and women. The slope values provided an additional distinguishing factor in male–female neck circumference relative to body size. Slope of the male regression was 0.31, close to the theoretical one-third (0.33) ratio of mass (x^3) to linear (x^1) dimensions [21]. At 0.27, the female regression slope did not maintain the theoretical ratio.

In contrast to the neck circumference by body weight plot, Fig. 3-5 illustrates male and female neck C7–tragus length against head circumference. Male and female data overlapped extensively. Regression slopes and R^2 were not different from zero. This plot clearly demonstrates that neck length and head circumference were poorly correlated.

Differences in Cervical Spine Morphology

Differences in cervical spine anatomical characteristics can change the method by which the cervical spine responds to head–neck inertial loading. This area received a considerable amount of attention in quantifying cervical spine anatomical characteristics. Differences in cervical

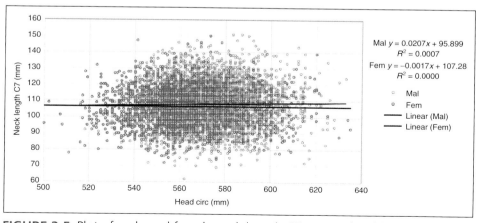

FIGURE 3-5 Plot of male and female neck length C7–tragus (mm) by head circumference (mm) with regression lines by sex. Male and female data overlap extensively. Regression slopes are not different from zero.

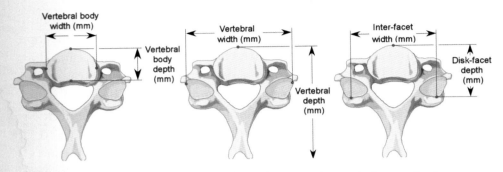

FIGURE 3-6 Cervical spine anatomical metrics were shown to be smaller in women across a number of studies. This may contribute to decreased stability of the cervical column and an increased risk of injury in women. (Used with permission from Stemper et al. [57].)

vertebral geometry between men and women were defined in a number of studies [16–18, 26, 29, 67]. In average-sized men and women, those studies identified smaller vertebral dimensions in women, focusing on vertebral body height and width, and overall vertebral depth (vertebral body to spinous process length). In a more recent study, Stemper and colleagues [57] reported metrics more relevant to mechanical stability in size-matched men and women (Fig. 3-6). The authors reasoned that dimensions such as the disk–facet depth, which quantified distance from the anterior aspect of the intervertebral disk to the posterior aspect of the facet joints, were more relevant to spinal stability. Interfacet width (lateral distance between facet joints) was also quantified. That study reported disk–facet depth and interfacet width were smaller in female volunteers compared to male volunteers size-matched based on head circumference. Head circumference is a meaningful metric as it correlates with head mass, which is important in head–neck inertial loading during rear impacts. The authors also demonstrated that a novel metric, the area of support, was smaller in that size-matched population of women (Fig. 3-7). Although column length was longer in the size-matched male population, the ratio of column length to support area, an assessment of cervical column slenderness, remained greater in women. This indicates that head circumference-matched female cervical spines are more slender and, therefore, more susceptible to bending during inertial loading of the head–neck complex. This

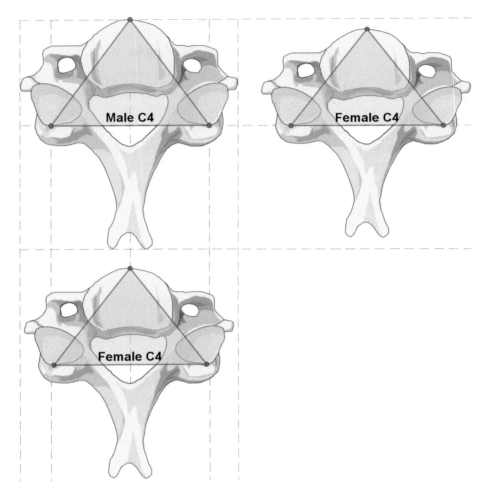

FIGURE 3-7 Cervical spines of women demonstrate a smaller area of support than those of men, possibly indicating less column stability and a greater likelihood of bending during external loads. (Used with permission from Stemper et al. [57].)

finding demonstrates that women are not simply "scaled down" men and that a fundamental difference exists in cervical spinal anatomy to predispose that population to increased injury risk during low velocity rear impacts.

Gender-based differences in cervical spine facet joint anatomical characteristics were also identified. Specifically, Yoganandan and colleagues [70] reported a 36% increased gap in cartilage coverage on the dorsal facet joint surface in women. The increased cartilage gap in women may expose the adjacent subchondral bone to direct stresses during loading experienced during rear impacts [8, 9, 37, 54]. Dorsal compression of the joint during the retraction phase [52] may damage bony structures or produce elevated stresses in the innervated subchondral bone, leading to nociceptive response. Decreased cartilage cover on the dorsal facet joint surface in women would predispose that population to pain mechanisms associated with whiplash-associated disorders [2].

Finally, anatomical variations in the superficial neck muscles may also contribute to differences between men and women in head–neck response to rear impacts. The neck muscles reflexively contract to stiffen the head–neck complex during rear impact, reducing spinal loads and preventing excessive soft tissue deformation that can lead to subcatastrophic or complete tissue failure [42]. Neck muscle precontraction in occupants aware of the impending impact decreased the likelihood of injury [25, 62] and the overall motion of the head–neck and cervical spine [44, 51]. However, the ability of reflexive contraction in the unaware occupant to stiffen the head–neck complex and protect the cervical spine remains unclear due to inherent delays in the neck muscle contraction scheme that may delay contraction and sufficient force buildup until after injury. It is acknowledged that soft tissue injury occurs within the first 100 ms following the impact. Reflex delay and electromechanical delay account for at least half of that and likely more [42, 60]. Following contraction onset, forces increase over time until reaching maximum contraction levels. Complicating the issue is that the vertically oriented neck muscles are not optimally positioned to affect inertial loading that occurs in the horizontal plane [4]. In other words, superficial neck muscle lines of action are oriented 90° away from the line of action for thoracic acceleration. Nonetheless, researchers have investigated this using human volunteers subjected to simulated rear impacts [4, 34] and computational modeling [60]. Those studies most often reported a marginal effect of reflexive neck muscle contraction, decreasing head–neck and spinal motions by a limited amount and offering limited protective effect for the occupant.

The level of cervical spine soft tissue protection offered through neck muscle precontraction or reflexive contraction depends on morphological characteristics. Muscle cross-sectional area is positively correlated with the magnitude of contractile force. Likewise, muscle centroid distance from the rotational axis (i.e., moment arm) determines the magnitude of bending moment applied to a joint during contraction. Neck muscle sizes were quantified using Upright MRI scans [47, 57] and normal supine MRI scans [13]. Stemper and colleagues [50] identified significantly decreased cross-sectional areas for anterior superficial neck muscles in women that likely indicate a decreased force-generating capacity (Fig. 3-8). That study also identified decreased moment arm distance in women. Those findings highlight that smaller female neck muscles produce less contractile force acting at a shorter distance away from the joint center and, therefore, have a lower capacity to affect intervertebral rotations and limit soft tissue distortions resulting in whiplash injuries. Those findings are supported by the work of Vasavada and colleagues [67, 68], who demonstrated lower neck muscle moment generating capacity in women, wherein female neck muscle strength was estimated to be only 71% of that of men.

This brief description of standard anthropometry, vertebral dimensions, and muscle size/positioning provides evidence of differing anthropometry between men and women. A female neck is not just a smaller version of a male neck; it is more slender, as noted by Vasavada and colleagues [67]. With larger muscles and vertebrae, men can better resist the fore and aft forces generated during rear impacts [48]. However, vertebra and muscle size are not the only terms in the equation of motion resistance. Cervical spine curvature also plays a part. Klinich and colleagues [30] reported wide variations of cervical curvature in an age- and gender-stratified sample of 180 adults. Lateral radiographs were obtained of seated volunteers looking straight ahead, and with heads flexed and extended. Twenty-seven landmarks were digitized on C1 and C2, and 18 landmarks on C3–C7. Midline Bézier curves were computed from landmarks obtained along the posterior margin of the vertebral bodies.

Neutral spine curvature index was 2.4%. Curvature angles less than 3% were relatively straight, and did not vary significantly between men and women. Relative to stature, curvature angle was invariant in men,

FIGURE 3-8
Smaller cross-sectional areas of superficial neck muscles in women produce less contractile force, and the muscles are positioned closer to the joint center across the cervical spine. Therefore, the ability of the neck muscles to influence dynamic cervical spine motions during low-velocity rear impacts is reduced.

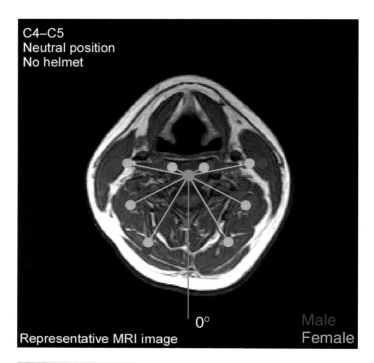

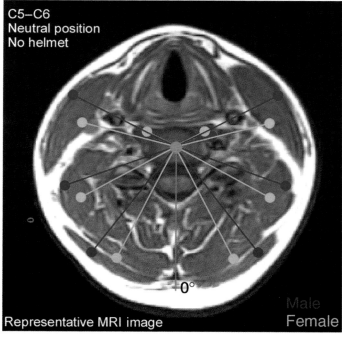

FIGURE 3.8
(*Continued*)

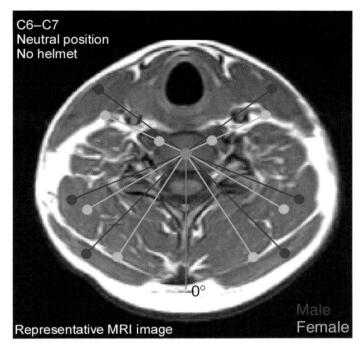

but decreased from 3.3% in shorter women to 2% in taller women. Neck length increased with stature in men and women (Fig. 3-9), although the correlation was low. A majority of volunteers (~86%) had midlordotic or superior lordotic curvature. Thirteen percent had straight curvature, and the rest had an inferior lordosis, kyphotic, or S-shaped Bézier curves.

Neck curvature influences muscle action. Vasavada and colleagues [67] described muscle wrapping around geometric objects in a neck muscle model, and found wrapping surfaces improved muscle path representation considerably. Further, Suderman and colleagues [63] demonstrated that kinematic linkage to cervical spine segments significantly affected neck flexion and extension simulation. Thus, representing neck curvature for correct muscle wrapping is important in accurate neck simulation.

This section has highlighted gender-based geometrical differences in neck and cervical spine anthropometry that may contribute to greater female susceptibility during low velocity automobile rear impacts. Anthropometry studies have shown that women have a larger head mass to

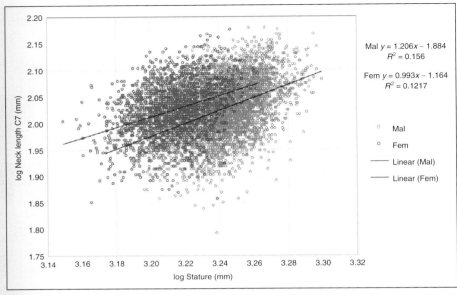

FIGURE 3-9 Log–log plot of C7–tragus neck length (mm) against stature (mm).

neck area ratio, which increases the severity of inertial loading on the cervical spine for a given automobile rear impact. Likewise, gender-based variations in cervical spine geometry may contribute to a more slender cervical column in women that is more likely to bend under an applied external load. Finally, studies incorporating magnetic resonance imaging have identified comparatively smaller neck muscle sizes in women and muscle centroids positioned closer to the joint center, indicating a reduced capacity of the superficial muscles to affect intervertebral rotations during dynamic loading of the head–neck complex. Each of these findings demonstrates that morphological differences in neck and cervical spine anatomy likely contribute to greater injury susceptibility of female occupants during low velocity rear impacts.

CONCLUSIONS

Women are historically vulnerable to injury during low velocity rear impacts. Clinical and experimental research supports this assertion. Explanations for increased susceptibility are highlighted in this chapter, and include morphological differences in body size relative to the seat, cervical curvature, cervical vertebrae, and neck muscles. Understanding these differences is key to improving automotive safety for women. Although automobiles were historically designed for the average size male, recognition of gender- and size-based differences has become apparent with adjustable and active head restraints, and the incorporation of small female crash test dummies in automotive safety assessments such as the New Car Assessment Program (NCAP) in the United States. Continuing to develop an understanding of biomechanically relevant morphological differences between men and women will help provide safer environments for all vehicle occupants.

REFERENCES

1. Aldman B. An analytical approach to the impact biomechanics of head and neck injury. 30th Annual Proceedings of the Association for the Advancement of Automotive Medicine. Montreal, Quebec; October 1986.

2. Bogduk N. On cervical zygapophysial joint pain after whiplash. Spine (Phila Pa 1976) 2011;36:S194–S199.

3. Bostrom O, Svensson MY, Aldman B, Hansson HA, Haaland Y, Loevsund P, Seeman T, Suneson A, Saeljoe A, Oertengren T. A new neck injury criterion candidate based on injury findings in the cervical spinal ganglia after experimental neck extension trauma. International IRCOBI Conference on the Biomechanics of Impact. Dublin, Ireland; September 1996.

4. Brault JR, Siegmund GP, Wheeler JB. Cervical muscle response during whiplash: evidence of a lengthening muscle contraction. Clin Biomech (Bristol, Avon) 2000;15:426–35.

5. Brault JR, Wheeler JB, Siegmund GP, Brault EJ. Clinical response of human subjects to rear-end automobile collisions. Arch Phys Med Rehabil 1998;79:72–80.

6. Carlsson A, Linder A, Davidsson J, Hell W, Schick S, Svensson M. Dynamic kinematic responses of female volunteers in rear impacts and comparison to previous male volunteer tests. Traffic Inj Prev 2011;12:347–57.

7. Cassidy JD, Carroll LJ, Cote P, Lemstra M, Berglund A, Nygren A. Effect of eliminating compensation for pain and suffering on the outcome of insurance claims for whiplash injury. N Engl J Med 2000;342:1179–86.

8. Cusick JF, Pintar FA, Yoganandan N. Whiplash syndrome: kinematic factors influencing pain patterns. Spine (Phila Pa 1976) 2001;26:1252–8.

9. Deng B, Begeman PC, Yang KH, Tashman S, King AI. Kinematics of human cadaver cervical spine during low speed rear-end impacts. Stapp Car Crash J 2000;44:171–88.

10. DeRosia J, Yoganandan N, Pintar FA. Rear impact responses of different sized adult Hybrid III dummies. Traffic Inj Prev 2004;5:50–5.

11. Dolinis J. Risk factors for "whiplash" in drivers: a cohort study of rear-end traffic crashes. Injury 1997;28:173–9.

12. Dwyer A, Aprill C, Bogduk N. Cervical zygapophyseal joint pain patterns. I: a study in normal volunteers. Spine (Phila Pa 1976) 1990;15:453–7.

13. Elliott JM, Jull GA, Noteboom JT, Durbridge GL, Gibbon WW. Magnetic resonance imaging study of cross-sectional area of the cervical extensor musculature in an asymptomatic cohort. Clin Anat 2007;20:35–40.

14. Eppinger R, Sun E, Kuppa S, Saul R. Supplement: development of improved injury criteria for the assessment of advanced automotive restraint systems-II. Washington, DC: National Highway Traffic Safety Administration; 2000.

15. Farmer CM, Wells JK, Lund AK. Effects of head restraint and seat redesign on neck injury risk in rear-end crashes. Traffic Inj Prev 2003;4:83–90.

16. Francis CC. Dimensions of the cervical vertebrae. Anat Rec 1955;122:603–9.

17. Frobin W, Leivseth G, Biggemann M, Brinckmann P. Vertebral height, disc height, posteroanterior displacement and dens-atlas gap in the cervical spine: precision measurement protocol and normal data. Clin Biomech (Bristol, Avon) 2002;17:423–31.

18. Gilad I, Nissan M. A study of vertebra and disc geometric relations of the human cervical and lumbar spine. Spine (Phila Pa 1976) 1986;11:154–7.

19. Gordon CC, Blackwell CL, Bradtmiller B, Parham JL, Barrientos P, Paquette SP, Corner BD, Carson JM, Venezia JC, Rockwell BM, et al. 2012 Anthropometric survey of U.S. Army personnel: methods and summary statistics. Natick, MA: Natick Soldier Research, Development and Engineering Center; 2014.

20. Gordon CC, Blackwell CL, Bradtmiller B, Parham JL, Hotzman J, Paquette SP, Corner BD, Hodge BM. 2010 Anthropometric survey of U.S. Marine Corps personnel: methods and summary statistics. Natick, MA: Natick Soldier Research, Development and Engineering Center; 2013.

21. Gould SJ. Allometry and size in ontogeny and phylogeny. Biol Rev Camb Philos Soc 1966;41:587–640.

22. Gould SJ. Geometric similarity in allometric growth: a contribution to the problem of scaling in the evolution of size. Am Nat 1971;105:113–36.

23. Grauer JN, Panjabi MM, Cholewicki J, Nibu K, Dvorak J. Whiplash produces an S-shaped curvature of the neck with hyperextension at lower levels. Spine (Phila Pa 1976) 1997;22:2489–94.

24. Hell W, Langwieder K, Walz F, Muser M, Krarner M, Hartwig E. Consequences for seat design due to rear end accident analysis, sled tests and possible test criteria for reducing cervical spine injuries after rear-end collision. International IRCOBI Conference on the Biomechanics of Impact. Sitges, Spain; September 1999.

25. Hendriks EJ, Scholten-Peeters GG, van der Windt DA, Neeleman-van der Steen CW, Oostendorp RA, Verhagen AP. Prognostic factors for poor recovery in acute whiplash patients. Pain 2005;114:408–16.

26. Hukuda S, Kojima Y. Sex discrepancy in the canal/body ratio of the cervical spine implicating the prevalence of cervical myelopathy in men. Spine (Phila Pa 1976) 2002;27:250–3.

27. Jakobsson L, Norin H, Svensson MY. Parameters influencing AIS 1 neck injury outcome in frontal impacts. Traffic Inj Prev 2004;5:156–63.

28. Jonsson B. Interaction between humans and car seats. Umea: Umea University; 2008.

29. Katz PR, Reynolds HM, Foust DR, Baum JK. Mid-sagittal dimensions of cervical vertebral bodies. Am J Phys Anthropol 1975;43:319–26.

30. Klinich KD, Ebert SM, Van Ee CA, Flannagan CA, Prasad M, Reed MP, Schneider LW. Cervical spine geometry in the automotive seated posture: variations with age, stature, and gender. Stapp Car Crash J 2004;48:301–30.

31. Linder A, Carlsson A, Svensson MY, Siegmund GP. Dynamic responses of female and male volunteers in rear impacts. Traffic Inj Prev 2008;9:592–9.

32. Linder A, Olsson T, Truedsson N, Morris A, Fildes B, Sparke L. Dynamic performances of different seat designs for low to medium velocity rear impact. Annu Proc Assoc Adv Automot Med 2001;45:187–201.

33. Luan F, Yang KH, Deng B, Begeman PC, Tashman S, King AI. Qualitative analysis of neck kinematics during low-speed rear-end impact. Clin Biomech (Bristol, Avon) 2000;15:649–57.

34. Magnusson ML, Pope MH, Hasselquist L, Bolte KM, Ross M, Goel VK, Lee JS, Spratt K, Clark CR, Wilder DG. Cervical electromyographic activity during low-speed rear impact. Eur Spine J 1999;8:118–25.

35. Ono K, Ejima S, Suzuki Y, Kaneoka K, Fukushima M, Ujihashi S. Prediction of neck injury risk based on the analysis of localized cervical vertebral motion of human volunteers during low-speed rear impacts. International IRCOBI Conference on the Biomechanics of Impact. Madrid, Spain; September 2006.

36. Pal GP, Routal RV, Saggu SK. The orientation of the articular facets of the zygapophyseal joints at the cervical and upper thoracic region. J Anat 2001;198:431–41.

37. Pearson AM, Ivancic PC, Ito S, Panjabi MM. Facet joint kinematics and injury mechanisms during simulated whiplash. Spine (Phila Pa 1976) 2004;29:390–7.

38. Penning L. Acceleration injury of the cervical spine by hypertranslation of the head, Part I: effect of normal translation of the head on cervical spine motion: a radiological study. Eur Spine J 1992;1:7–12.

39. Penning L. Acceleration injury of the cervical spine by hypertranslation of the head, Part II: effect of hypertranslation of the head on cervical spine motion: discussion of literature data. Eur Spine J 1992;1:13–9.

40. Richter M, Otte D, Pohlemann T, Krettek C, Blauth M. Whiplash-type neck distortion in restrained car drivers: frequency, causes and long-term results. Eur Spine J 2000;9:109–17.

41. Schmitt KU, Muser MH, Walz FH, Niederer PF. Nkm—a proposal for a neck protection criterion for low-speed rear-end impacts. Traffic Inj Prev 2002;3:117–26.

42. Siegmund GP, Brault JR, Chimich DD. Do cervical muscles play a role in whiplash injury? J Whiplash Relat Disord 2002;1:23–40.

43. Siegmund GP, Myers BS, Davis MB, Bohnet HF, Winkelstein BA. Mechanical evidence of cervical facet capsule injury during whiplash: a cadaveric study using combined shear, compression, and extension loading. Spine (Phila Pa 1976) 2001;26:2095–101.

44. Siegmund GP, Sanderson DJ, Myers BS, Inglis JT. Awareness affects the response of human subjects exposed to a single whiplash-like perturbation. Spine (Phila Pa 1976) 2003;28:671–9.

45. Sokal RR, Rohlf FJ. Biometry: the principles and practice of statistics in biological research. 3rd ed. New York, NY: W. H. Freeman and Co; 1995.

46. States JD, Balcerak JC, Williams JS, Morris AT, Babcock W, Polvino R, Riger P, Dawley RE. Injury frequency and head restraint effectiveness in rear-end impact accidents. 16th Stapp Car Crash Conference. New York, NY; November 1972. pp. 228–45.

47. Stemper BD, Baisden JL, Yoganandan N, Pintar FA, Paskoff GR, Shender BS. Determination of normative neck muscle morphometry using upright MRI with comparison to supine data. Aviat Space Environ Med 2010;81:878–82.

48. Stemper BD, Derosia JJ, Yoganan N, Pintar FA, Shender BS, Paskoff GR. Gender dependent cervical spine anatomical differences in size-matched volunteers—biomed 2009. Biomed Sci Instrum 2009;45:149–54.

49. Stemper BD, Storvik SG. Incorporation of lower neck shear forces to predict facet joint injury risk in low-speed automotive rear impacts. Traffic Inj Prev 2010;11:300–8.

50. Stemper BD, Yoganandan N, Baisden JL, Pintar FA, Shender BS, Paskoff G. Biomechanical implications of gender-dependent muscle locations. 2008 ASME Summer Bioengineering Conference. Marco Island, FL; June 2008.

51. Stemper BD, Yoganandan N, Cusick JF, Pintar FA. Stabilizing effect of precontracted neck musculature in whiplash. Spine (Phila Pa 1976) 2006;31:E733–E738.

52. Stemper BD, Yoganandan N, Gennarelli TA, Pintar FA. Localized cervical facet joint kinematics under physiological and whiplash loading. J Neurosurg Spine 2005;3:471–6.

53. Stemper BD, Yoganandan N, Pintar FA. Gender dependent cervical spine segmental kinematics during whiplash. J Biomech 2003;36:1281–9.

54. Stemper BD, Yoganandan N, Pintar FA. Gender- and region-dependent local facet joint kinematics in rear impact: implications in whiplash injury. Spine (Phila Pa 1976) 2004;29:1764–71.

55. Stemper BD, Yoganandan N, Pintar FA. Effect of head restraint backset on head-neck kinematics in whiplash. Accid Anal Prev 2006;38:317–23.

56. Stemper BD, Yoganandan N, Pintar FA, Maiman DJ. The relationship between lower neck shear force and facet joint kinematics during automotive rear impacts. Clin Anat 2011;24:319–26.

57. Stemper BD, Yoganandan N, Pintar FA, Maiman DJ, Meyer MA, DeRosia J, Shender BS, Paskoff G. Anatomical gender differences in cervical vertebrae of size-matched volunteers. Spine (Phila Pa 1976) 2008;33:E44–E49.

58. Stemper BD, Yoganandan N, Pintar FA, Rao RD. Anterior longitudinal ligament injuries in whiplash may lead to cervical instability. Med Eng Phys 2006;28:515–24.

59. Stemper BD, Yoganandan N, Rao RD, Pintar FA. Influence of thoracic ramping on whiplash kinematics. Clin Biomech (Bristol, Avon) 2005;20:1019–28.

60. Stemper BD, Yoganandan N, Rao RD, Pintar FA. Reflex muscle contraction in the unaware occupant in whiplash injury. Spine (Phila Pa 1976) 2005;30:2794–8; discussion 2799.

61. Storvik SG, Stemper BD, Yoganandan N, Pintar FA. Population-based estimates of whiplash injury using NASS CDS data—biomed 2009. Biomed Sci Instrum 2009;45:244–9.

62. Sturzenegger M, DiStefano G, Radanov BP, Schnidrig A. Presenting symptoms and signs after whiplash injury: the influence of accident mechanisms. Neurology 1994;44:688–93.

63. Suderman BL, Krishnamoorthy B, Vasavada AN. Neck muscle paths and moment arms are significantly affected by wrapping surface parameters. Comput Methods Biomech Biomed Engin 2012;15:735–44.

64. Svensson MY, Aldman B, Hansson HA, Lövsund P, Seeman T, Suneson A, Örtengren T. Pressure effects in the spinal canal during whiplash extension motion: a possible cause of injury to the cervical spinal ganglia. International IRCOBI Conference on the Biomechanics of Impact. Eindhoven, The Netherlands; September 1993.

65. Szabo TJ, Welcher JB, Anderson RD. Human occupant kinematic response to low-speed rear end impacts. 38th Stapp Car Crash Conference. Fort Lauderdale, FL; 1994.

66. Tencer AF, Mirza S, Bensel K. Internal loads in the cervical spine during motor vehicle rear-end impacts: the effect of acceleration and head-to-head restraint proximity. Spine (Phila Pa 1976) 2002;27:34–42.

67. Vasavada AN, Danaraj J, Siegmund GP. Head and neck anthropometry, vertebral geometry and neck strength in height-matched men and women. J Biomech 2008;41:114–21.

68. Vasavada AN, Li S, Delp SL. Influence of muscle morphometry and moment arms on the moment-generating capacity of human neck muscles. Spine (Phila Pa 1976) 1998;23:412–22.

69. Viano DC. Seat influences on female neck responses in rear crashes: a reason why women have higher whiplash rates. Traffic Inj Prev 2003;4:228–39.

70. Yoganandan N, Knowles SA, Maiman DJ, Pintar FA. Anatomic study of the morphology of human cervical facet joint. Spine (Phila Pa 1976) 2003;28:2317–23.

71. Yoganandan N, Pintar FA, Stemper BD, Schlick MB, Philippens M, Wismans J. Biomechanics of human occupants in simulated rear crashes: documentation of neck injuries and comparison of injury criteria. Stapp Car Crash J 2000;44:189–204.

CHAPTER 4

Reorganized Motor and Sensorimotor Control in Whiplash

Implications for Training

Deborah Falla and Gwendolen Jull

Whiplash-associated disorders (WAD) are a significant public health problem. Approximately 50% of those affected report persistent disability more than 1 year after the injury, resulting in both substantial personal and societal costs [4]. Moreover, up to 30% of those affected will remain moderately to severely disabled. The physical and psychological features associated with WAD are diverse, and various factors may contribute to the chronicity of symptoms. Here, the focus is on the motor and sensorimotor adaptations that may occur following a whiplash injury. Moreover, the implications of these findings for the rehabilitation of people with WAD are discussed.

MOTOR AND SENSORIMOTOR ADAPTATIONS

Individuals who have suffered a whiplash injury typically present with some degree of impaired motor function such as reduced neck strength, which may be apparent around all axes, and/or reduced force steadiness. Range of motion is also usually restricted and, in general, people with neck pain may show increased range of motion variability, decreased movement speed, and reduced smoothness of neck movement (for review see [17]).

Although pain can impair motor output, several studies have shown that in the presence of goal-oriented submaximal tasks, the kinematic output may be unchanged [15]. Muscular adaptation occurs (i.e., redistribution of the activity within the same muscle or across synergistic muscles) to maintain unaltered motor output but with modified muscle load. Accordingly, changes in muscle activation and muscle coordination are well documented in people with whiplash-induced neck pain and are largely similar to the changes observed in people with insidious-onset neck pain. Such changes may include reduced activation of the deep cervical flexors (longus colli, longus capitis) during performance of brief isometric craniocervical flexion contractions [9] or delayed activation of these muscles when exposed to rapid postural perturbations [8]. Poorer control of the deep cervical flexor muscles is associated with increased activation (likely compensatory) of the sternocleidomastoid and anterior scalene muscles [9], an observation that has been documented within the first 4 weeks of a whiplash injury [32]. More recent work also showed reduced activation of the deep extensor muscle, semispinalis cervicis, in people with trauma-induced neck pain [30], reinforcing the frequent observation of impaired activation of the deeper spinal muscles in people with spinal pain disorders.

Reduced specificity of neck muscle activation is another feature of altered motor control of the neck observed in people with chronic neck pain disorders [12, 30] (Fig. 4-1). A loss of the predefined patterns of muscle activation has been noted for several neck muscles (e.g., sternocleidomastoid, splenius capitis, semispinalis cervicis) in several patient groups (e.g., WAD, idiopathic neck pain) and supports the relatively consistent finding of augmented activity of the superficial muscles in people with neck pain disorders, regardless of the task examined; for example, cervical flexion, craniocervical flexion, and movements of the upper limb. Increased coactivation of the neck flexor and extensor muscles may also be present, and is inversely correlated with total neck strength and positively correlated with levels of pain and perceived disability [23]. High levels of neck muscle coactivation may reflect an

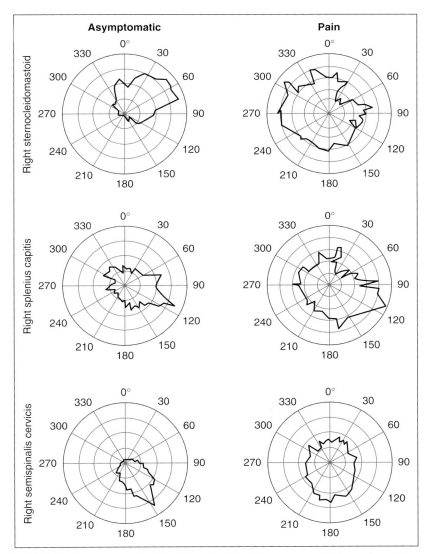

FIGURE 4-1 Representative directional activation curves obtained from the sternocleidomastoid, splenius capitis and semispinalis cervicis muscles during a circular contraction performed at 15 Newtons presented for a control subject and a patient with chronic neck pain. Note the defined activation of the sterno-cleidomastoid, splenius capitis, and semispinalis cervicis for the control subject with minimal activity during the antagonist phase of the task. Conversely, the directional activation curves for the patient indicate more even activation levels of each muscle for all directions resulting in increased coactivation of the neck flexor and extensor muscles. (Reprinted with permission from Falla et al. [12], Lindstrøm et al. [23] and Schomacher et al. [30].)

attempt to voluntarily increase the stability of the head/neck for the fear of performing potentially painful movements. This fits with the contemporary theory that sensorimotor adaptation to pain has a general aim (at least in the short term) to protect the painful/threatened body part from real or anticipated further pain/injury [16].

Recent work has revealed that during repetitive arm movements, load sharing between neck muscles, as seen in asymptomatic people, is reduced in people with WAD. That is, people with WAD showed less variability in the pattern of neck muscle activation throughout the repetitive task [29]. Decreased motor variability during repetitive work has also been reported in people with chronic neck–shoulder pain and may result in higher fatigue and pain. Studies in patients with trapezius myalgia show similar results. For example, patients with trapezius myalgia activate the same region of the upper trapezius muscle continuously throughout a sustained shoulder abduction contraction, whereas asymptomatic subjects show redistribution of muscle activity across the duration of the contraction, resulting in less muscle fatigue [6].

Whiplash-induced pain has also been associated with a number of sensorimotor adaptations including impaired proprioception, reduced postural stability, and reduced smoothness of eye movements. Greater errors in positioning the head following voluntary movement have been shown in persons with neck pain of both insidious and traumatic onset, but proprioceptive acuity appears to be more affected in people with chronic whiplash especially in those reporting higher pain and disability and dizziness [34]. In addition to greater repositioning errors with head movement, some people with WAD show reduced proprioception at the shoulder and elbow that could affect the coordination and movement of their upper limb. Disturbed postural stability includes larger postural trunk sway both in stance tasks and in complex tasks such as walking up and down stairs, and reduced head stability in response to predictable and unpredictable postural perturbations [25]. Consistent with observations for head relocation accuracy, people with whiplash-induced pain generally show greater disturbances compared to patients with idiopathic neck pain, and postural instability is positively associated with the symptom of dizziness [34]. Changes in oculomotor control have also been demonstrated in people with whiplash, suggestive of disturbances in the cervicocollic and cervico-ocular reflexes [34].

Variability of Motor and Sensorimotor Adaptations

As reviewed above, people with WAD may present with many motor and/or sensorimotor adaptations (Fig. 4-2). However, it is well known that people with WAD form a heterogeneous group in terms of the associated pain mechanisms, psychological features, and physical signs. In relation to the type and extent of neuromuscular adaptations observed in people with WAD, there is substantial variability between individual patients. This variability likely relates to interactions between the nature and extent of the injury, the magnitude of pain and disability, and the

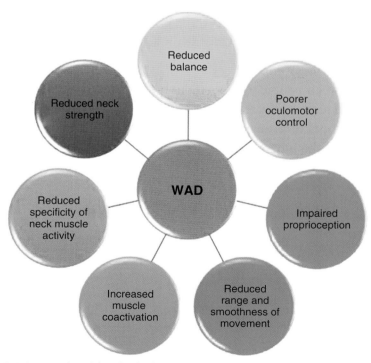

FIGURE 4-2 People with whiplash-associated disorders (WAD) may present with many motor and sensorimotor disturbances that may include, but that are not limited to, those presented here.

presence and magnitude of attendant stress reactions. Some evidence supports the premise that variability is partially related to the magnitude of pain. For example, augmented sternocleidomastoid and anterior scalene muscle activity during repetitive arm movements is greatest in patients reporting higher levels of pain and disability [7]. Furthermore, higher levels of pain are associated with greater delays in the activation of the deep cervical flexors during rapid flexion of the shoulder and lower amplitude of activation during isometric craniocervical flexion [13].

We recently examined the effects of experimentally induced neck muscle pain on multimuscle control of neck movements during an aiming task [15]. A general decrease in the electromyography (EMG) amplitude was observed in the injected muscle together with redistribution (decrease/increase) of the activation of other muscles, in a subject-specific manner. Thus, this work showed that people tend to adopt an individual control strategy so that a painful stimulus in the neck triggers a subject-specific redistribution of neck muscular activation (Fig. 4-3). These findings support the proposal of a heterogeneous adaptation of motor control in response to pain [16].

Similar to motor adaptations, sensorimotor disturbances are variable between people with WAD in both the nature of impairments and their frequency of presentation [34]. All or any one combination of disturbances in proprioception, balance, and oculomotor control may present in the individual.

IMPLICATIONS FOR TRAINING

This section provides an overview of key principles underlying prescription of therapeutic exercise for neck pain disorders, including WAD, as informed by the research into neuromuscular adaptations in association with neck pain.

Specificity of Exercise

Significant reductions in pain and disability have been observed for various types of training programs in patients with neck pain including

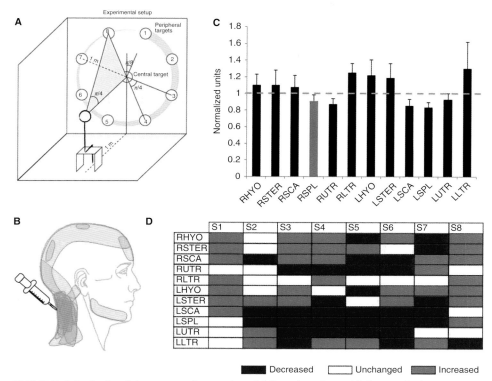

FIGURE 4-3 **A:** Participants performed multidirectional, multiplanar aiming movements of the head. Nine circular targets (one "central target" plus 8 "peripheral targets") were placed on a whitewall following a circular trajectory. Participants wore a helmet mounted with laser pointers, and the task consisted of moving their head and neck to aim laser pointers from the central target to each peripheral target following the tempo provided by a metronome. Electromyography (EMG) was recorded from multiple neck muscles. **B:** The task was completed at baseline (no pain) and immediately following the injection of hypertonic saline into the right splenius capitis muscle (pain). **C:** Mean and SD of the EMG amplitude recorded for each muscle in the painful condition normalized relative to the baseline condition. The gray dotted line indicates the level of activity that would be comparable between conditions. The injected muscle, the right splenius capitis, is highlighted in red; note the overall decreased activity of this muscle. Other muscles showed either an increase or decrease of activity across all subjects. **D:** Individual data for each of the eight subjects showing the direction of change in EMG amplitude of each muscle between the baseline and the painful condition. Red indicates an increase of EMG amplitude in the painful condition compared to baseline, blue indicates decreased EMG amplitude, and white indicates no change. Note the individual specific patterns of modulation of EMG amplitude. No two subjects showed the same strategy. (R, Right and L, Left; HYO, Sterno Hyoideus; STER, Sternocleidomastoideus; SCA, Anterior Scalenus; SPL, Splenius Capitis; UTR, Upper trapezius; LTR, Lower Trapezius). (Data from Gizzi et al. [15].)

low-intensity and high-intensity training. Thus, various training approaches may be appropriate for relief of pain. However, patients may respond to different exercise protocols, depending on the stage of their disorder and factors such as their level of pain, disability, and degree of neuromuscular impairment. For example, there is evidence that gentle low load exercise produces a superior immediate hypoalgesic effect than higher load exercise [27] (Fig. 4-4). Accordingly, low load exercise appears to be a better approach to management in the initial stages of rehabilitation when pain is the primary problem for the patient. Furthermore, specific motor control training can change control of the deep and superficial muscles in neck pain. For instance, targeted training of the deep cervical flexors increases their activation during an isometric

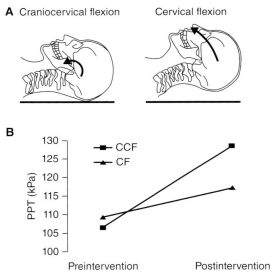

FIGURE 4-4 A: Patients with chronic neck pain were randomized into two training groups. The craniocervical flexion exercise involves a gentle nodding movement of the head such that it remains in contact with the supporting surface, flexion motion occurring predominantly about the upper cervical motion segments. In contrast, the head is lifted off the supporting surface during the cervical flexion exercise, and flexion occurs predominantly about the lower cervical motion segments. **B:** Change in pressure pain threshold recorded over the most symptomatic cervical motion segment immediately following one session (~3 minute) of exercise. Note the significantly increased pressure pain threshold (reduced pain sensitivity). (Reprinted with permission from O'Leary et al. [27].)

task [18], improves the speed of their activation when challenged by postural perturbations [14, 18], and enhances the degree of directional specificity of neck muscle activity during multidirectional isometric contractions of the neck [11]. Activity of superficial neck muscles can also be reduced with specific motor control training [18], even after a single session [24]. Importantly, deep muscle control does not appear to be changed by generic forms of exercise [18]. In contrast, exercise programs utilizing higher load endurance and strength protocols have shown superior gains in cervical muscle strength, endurance, and re-sistance to fatigue compared to low load programs [10, 28]. Taken to-gether, these findings highlight the need for specificity in the approach to therapeutic exercise prescription for people with neck pain, and con-firm that specific neuronal, muscle, and functional changes in motor output in response to exercise adaptations to training are specific to the mode of exercise [1]. Accordingly, it is generally recommended that exercise programs for patients with neck pain are based on a precise assessment of neuromuscular function and are progressed from lower load to higher load exercises [19].

In relation to sensorimotor control, management of symptoms such as dizziness and unsteadiness whiplash injury includes addressing the many potential causes of altered cervical afferent input such as atten-tion to pain, inflammation, stress, neuromuscular adaptations, as well as addressing the adaptive changes in the sensorimotor system [34]. Symptomatic relief has been obtained with a number of modalities, in-cluding specific exercise such as retraining joint position sense, manual therapy, and acupuncture. Nevertheless, adaptive changes in the senso-rimotor system appear to be better targeted with direct training of the impairment, for example, training balance, joint position sense, move-ment sense, or eye movement control.

Early Rehabilitation

Changes in neuromuscular control appear early following a whiplash trauma [32]. In addition, experimental pain studies indicate that pain has an immediate effect on the behavior of the neck muscles, simi-lar to that seen in people with chronic neck pain [3]. It is therefore suggested that exercise to address motor and sensorimotor adaptations is commenced early [19]. The gentle low load motor control exercises to restore deep muscle control can be undertaken safely and in a non-provocative manner in these early stages as can some of the interventions for sensorimotor control such as simple balance training.

The benefit of early rehabilitation of motor and sensorimotor control has not been fully examined in clinical trials. Nevertheless, failure to rehabilitate altered motor control may result in further long-term adaptations including changes in muscle structural properties. For instance, the presence of fatty tissue infiltration of the extensor muscle group, which is seen in patients with moderate to severe pain following a whiplash injury, is not detected until 3 months after the injury [5]. Potentially, such structural changes may, at least partially, represent a long- term consequence of altered motor control (e.g., muscle disuse) and may be prevented by specific and early training interventions.

Pain-Free Exercise

Exercises that cause pain can reinforce altered motor behavior and, importantly, inhibit the process of motor relearning [2]. Thus the type, load, and frequency of exercise should be tailored toward the patient to ensure that exercise can be performed in a pain-free manner. In the initial stages of rehabilitation, the dosage of exercise prescribed should reflect a volume that permits stimulus of muscle performance but remains short of symptom reproduction. In effect, gentle low load exercise produces an immediate hypoalgesic effect [27]. Therefore, appropriate exercise may be used to help provide immediate pain relief for the patient. Higher load exercise did not produce an immediate hypoalgesic effect, which further demonstrates that gentle and specific exercise is a superior approach to management in the initial stages of rehabilitation when pain is a key issue. As rehabilitation is gradually progressed over time to a dosage reflecting higher load strength and endurance, monitoring of patients' symptoms is recommended to ensure that any discomfort experienced during exercise associated with fatigue is not sustained between sessions.

Variable Response to Training

People with persistent WAD form a heterogeneous group with variable and sometimes complex patterns of coexisting physical and psychological impairments [31]. Thus, it is reasonable to expect that not all patients would benefit from the same intervention and that some may not benefit from exercise at all. This premise is supported by randomized controlled trials on exercise for chronic WAD that have shown large variability in patient outcome [22, 26, 33]. Similar variability in outcome is observed in people with idiopathic neck pain. The potential physiological mechanisms underlying the individual whiplash patient's pain appear to moderate the effect of exercise. This was revealed in a clinical trial testing the effect of a specific rehabilitation program on individuals with chronic WAD [20]. Persons with initial higher levels of pain and disability in association with widespread mechanical and cold hyperalgesia (suggesting the presence of augmented central pain processing mechanisms, loss of descending inhibition, or a neuropathic pain state; 25% of the cohort) were not as responsive to the rehabilitation program in terms of reduction in pain and disability and improvement in motor control. In contrast, individuals who sought treatment for widespread mechanical hyperalgesia only or without abnormal sensory features were more responsive to the exercise program (Fig. 4-5).

Recent work highlights that exercise interventions are more effective when targeted to findings of a detailed assessment and that people with features consistent with nociceptive pain (e.g., features of pain that imply a proportional and predictable relationship to mechanical loading) are more likely to respond favorably. Furthermore, the degree of muscle impairment present in the individual before the commencement of training may be an important determinant of symptom relief. This hypothesis was supported by a study that showed that specific training of the deep cervical flexor muscles in patients with chronic neck pain reduces pain and increases the activation of these muscles, especially in patients with the poorest activation of their deep cervical flexors prior to training [14]. Taken together, these findings suggest that the selection of exercise based on a precise assessment of the

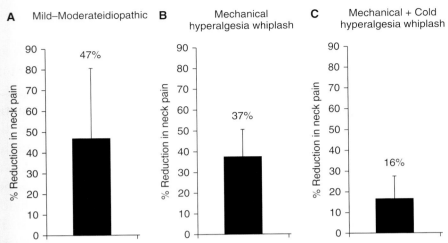

FIGURE 4-5 Mean and SD of the percent reduction in neck pain intensity reported following a rehabilitation program, including specific exercise, for individuals with chronic whiplash-associated disorders (WAD) and people with idiopathic neck pain. Note a 47% reduction in neck pain after 6 weeks of specific exercise in a group of patients with mild/moderate idiopathic neck pain (data from Falla et al. [10].) An 8-week rehabilitation program including the same specific exercises resulted in a 37% reduction in neck pain intensity in people with WAD with signs of mechanical hyperalgesia (data from Jull et al. [20].) The response to the same intervention was only 16% in people with WAD with signs of widespread mechanical and cold hyperalgesia (data from Jull et al. [20].) Thus, response to exercise is highly variable in people with neck pain disorders, and the effect of exercise may be moderated by other factors such as central sensitization.

patients' neuromuscular control, and targeted exercise interventions based on this assessment are likely to be the most beneficial to patients with neck pain.

Predicting Response to Training

A recent study on patients with chronic WAD showed a greater reduction in neck pain and neck-related disability after 3 and 6 months, following a neck-specific exercise program, with or without the addition of a behavioral approach, compared to the prescription of general physical activity [22]. Although significant improvements were observed for the neck-specific training groups, as expected, there were both responders and nonresponders to treatment in all groups. Subsequently, we evaluated whether the type of exercise intervention is a determinant of clinically important neck disability or pain reduction in chronic WAD, and whether features of the patient's baseline presentation were associated with outcome following exercise interventions [21]. The only significant factor associated with a reduction of both neck pain and neck-related disability at 3 and 12 months was participation in the neck-specific exercise program. Patients allocated to this group had up to 5.3 times higher odds of achieving disability reduction, and 3.9 times higher odds of achieving pain reduction compared to those in the physical activity group. The absence of dizziness was a factor associated with reduction in neck disability, increasing the odds 4.5 times. The symptom of dizziness has been associated with many sensorimotor disturbances in people with chronic WAD including impaired balance, proprioception deficits, and disturbances of oculomotor control [34]. Thus, very likely, patients with dizziness require a specific intervention also targeting those features of sensorimotor control and not only neck-specific exercise that was employed in this study. Psychological factors were not associated with either outcome, which is consistent with a recent observation that the degree of psychological distress did not modify the effect of treatment in chronic WAD [26].

CONCLUSIONS

Many factors can contribute to disturbed motor and sensorimotor function in the whiplash-injured patient including the nature of injury, pain, and associated psychological distress. These factors not only contribute to the responses in the neuromuscular system but they can moderate the effect of exercise. Although programs of supervised exercise may provide a clinical benefit to some patients in both the short and the long term, the response to exercise is highly variable, with responses ranging from excellent outcome to no relevant benefit. People who respond well are likely to be individuals in whom peripheral nociceptive input is continuing to drive their experience of pain. In contrast, it is important to recognize that people who do not respond as well to exercise interventions may have other causes also driving their pain experience, for example, central sensitization, injury/pathology severity. Thus, although it is unquestionable that sensorimotor control is affected, a goal is to identify individuals who will benefit most from rehabilitation of motor and sensorimotor function. Further research may also inform more effective exercise strategies.

REFERENCES

1. Adkins D, Boychuk J, Remple M, Kleim J. Motor training induces experience-specific patterns of plasticity across motor cortex and spinal cord. J Appl Physiol 2006; 101:1776–82.

2. Boudreau S, Romaniello A, Wang K, Svensson P, Sessle BJ, Arendt-Nielsen L. The effects of intra-oral pain on motor cortex neuroplasticity associated with short-term novel tongue-protrusion training in humans. Pain 2007;132:169–78.

3. Cagnie B, Dirks R, Schouten M, Parlevliet T, Cambier D, Danneels L. Functional reorganization of cervical flexor activity because of induced muscle pain evaluated by muscle functional magnetic resonance imaging. Man Ther 2011;16(5):470–5.

4. Carroll LJ, Holm LW, Hogg-Johnson S, Côtè P, Cassidy JD, Haldeman S, Nordin M, Hurwitz EL, Carragee EJ, van der Velde G, et al. Course and prognostic factors for neck pain in whiplash-associated disorders (WAD): results of the Bone and Joint Decade 2000–2010 Task Force on Neck Pain and Its Associated Disorders. Spine (Phila Pa 1976) 2008;33:S83–S92.

5. Elliott J, Pedler A, Kenardy J, Galloway G, Jull G, Sterling M. The temporal development of fatty infiltrates in the neck muscles following whiplash injury: an association with pain and posttraumatic stress. PLoS One 2011;6(6):e21194.

6. Falla D, Andersen H, Danneskiold-Samsøe B, Arendt-Nielsen L, Farina D. Adaptations of upper trapezius muscle activity during sustained contractions in women with fibromyalgia. J Electromyogr Kinesiol 2010;20(3):457–64.

7. Falla D, Bilenkij G, Jull G. Patients with chronic neck pain demonstrate altered patterns of muscle activation during performance of a functional upper limb task. Spine 2004;29(13):1436–40.

8. Falla D, Jull G, Hodges PW. Feedforward activity of the cervical flexor muscles during voluntary arm movements is delayed in chronic neck pain. Exp Brain Res 2004; 157:43–48.

9. Falla D, Jull G, Hodges PW. Patients with neck pain demonstrate reduced electromyographic activity of the deep cervical flexor muscles during performance of the cranio-cervical flexion test. Spine 2004;29(19):2108–14.

10. Falla D, Jull G, Hodges P, Vicenzino B. An endurance-strength training regime is effective in reducing myoelectric manifestations of cervical flexor muscle fatigue in females with chronic neck pain. Clin Neurophysiol 2006;117:828–37.

11. Falla D, Lindstrøm R, Rechter L, Boudreau S, Petzke F. Effectiveness of an 8-week exercise programme on pain and specificity of neck muscle activity in patients with chronic neck pain: a randomized controlled study. Eur J Pain 2013;17:1517–28.

12. Falla D, Lindstrøm R, Rechter L, Farina D. Effect of pain on the modulation in discharge rate of sternocleidomastoid motor units with force direction. Clin Neurophysiol 2010;121:744–53.

13. Falla D, O'Leary S, Farina D, Jull G. Association between intensity of pain and impairment in onset and activation of the deep cervical flexors in patients with persistent neck pain. Clin J Pain 2011;27(4):309–14.

14. Falla D, O'Leary S, Farina D, Jull G. The change in deep cervical flexor activity after training is associated with the degree of pain reduction in patients with chronic neck pain. Clin J Pain 2012;28(7):628–34.

15. Gizzi L, Muceli S, Petzke F, Falla D. Experimental muscle pain impairs the synergistic modular control of neck muscles. PLoS One in press.

16. Hodges PW, Tucker K. Moving differently in pain: a new theory to explain the adaptation to pain. Pain 2011;152:S90–S98.

17. Jull G. Considerations in the physical rehabilitation of patients with whiplash-associated disorders. Spine (Phila Pa 1976) 2011;36:S286–S291.

18. Jull G, Falla D, Vicenzino B, Hodges PW. The effect of therapeutic exercise on activation of the deep cervical flexor muscles in people with chronic neck pain. Man Ther 2009;14:696–701.

19. Jull G, Sterling M, Falla D, Treleaven J, O'Leary S. Whiplash, headache and neck pain: research based directions for physical therapies. Edinburgh: Elsevier, Churchill Livingstone; 2008.

20. Jull G, Sterling M, Kenardy J, Beller E. Does the presence of sensory hypersensitivity influence outcomes of physical rehabilitation for chronic whiplash?—a preliminary RCT. Pain 2007;129:28–34.

21. Landén Ludvigsson M, Petersen G, Dedering A, Falla D, Peolsson A. Factors associated with pain and disability reduction following exercise interventions in chronic whiplash. Eur J Pain in press.

22. Landén Ludvigsson M, Peterson G, O'Leary S, Dedering Å, Peolsson A. The effect of neck-specific exercise with, or without a behavioral approach, on pain, disability, and

self-efficacy in chronic whiplash-associated disorders: a randomized clinical trial. Clin J Pain 2014;31:294–303.

23. Lindstrøm R, Schomacher J, Farina D, Rechter L, Falla D. Association between neck muscle co-activation, pain, and strength in women with neck pain. Man Ther 2011;16(1):80–6.

24. Lluch E, Schomacher J, Gizzi L, Petzke F, Seegar D, Falla D. Immediate effects of active cranio-cervical flexion exercise versus passive mobilisation of the upper cervical spine on pain and performance on the cranio-cervical flexion test. Man Ther 2014;19(1):25–31.

25. Michaelson P, Michaelson M, Jaric S, Latash ML, Sjolander P, Djupsjobacka M. Vertical posture and head stability in patients with chronic neck pain. J Rehabil Med 2003;35(5):229–35.

26. Michaleff ZA, Maher CG, Lin CW, Rebbeck T, Jull G, Latimer J, Connelly L, Sterling M. Comprehensive physiotherapy exercise programme or advice for chronic whiplash (PROMISE): a pragmatic randomised controlled trial. Lancet 2014;384:133–41.

27. O'Leary S, Falla D, Hodges P, Jull G, Vicenzino B. Specific therapeutic exercise of the neck induces immediate local hypoalgesia. J Pain 2007;8:832–9.

28. O'Leary S, Jull G, Kim M, Uthaikhup S, Vicenzino B. Training mode-dependent changes in motor performance in neck pain. Arch Phys Med Rehabil 2012;93(7):1225–33.

29. Peterson G, Nilsson D, Trygg J, et al. Novel insights into the interplay between ventral neck muscles in individuals with whiplash-associated disorders. Under Review.

30. Schomacher J, Farina D, Lindstroem R, Falla D. Chronic trauma-induced neck pain impairs the neural control of the deep semispinalis cervicis muscle. Clin Neurophysiol 2012;123(7):1403–8.

31. Sterling M, Jull G, Vicenzino B, Kenardy J. Sensory hypersensitivity occurs soon after whiplash injury and is associated with poor recovery. Pain 2003;104:509–17.

32. Sterling M, Jull G, Vicenzino B, Kenardy J, Darnell R. Development of motor dysfunction following whiplash injury. Pain 2003;103:65–73.

33. Stewart MJ, Maher CG, Refshauge KM, Herbert RD, Bogduk N, Nicholas M. Randomized controlled trial of exercise for chronic whiplash-associated disorders. Pain 2007;128:59–68.

34. Treleaven J. Dizziness, unsteadiness, visual disturbances, and postural control: implications for the transition to chronic symptoms after a whiplash trauma. Spine (Phila Pa 1976) 2011;36:S211–S217.

CHAPTER 5

Trigeminal Pain and Sensitization
Proposal of a New Stochastic Model

Peter Svensson and Abhishek Kumar

I n this chapter, we will discuss the complex relationship between cervical pain related to whiplash trauma and pain in the trigeminal (V) region. We will specifically focus on the painful temporomandibular disorders (TMD) and start with a brief review of the clinical observations of overlaps between TMD pain and cervical pain. Then we summarize what is known about V sensitization and discuss possible mechanisms that may account for such overlaps in symptom presentation. In the last part, we will report on purported risk factors for TMD pain and finally propose a new stochastic model to account for complex interactions between cervical pain and V pain and sensitization.

CLINICAL PRESENTATIONS

A typical presentation of pain patterns in a patient with V pain and cervical pain and a history of a whiplash trauma 3 years previously is shown in Fig. 5-1. The patient experiences an almost constant and daily pain both in the jaws and in the neck that is exacerbated by physical function such as chewing and turning the head. The pain is also

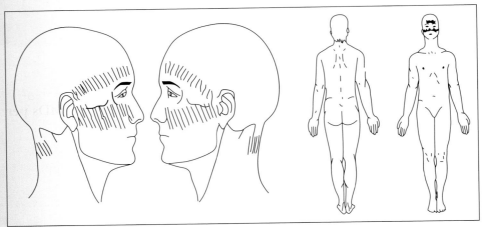

FIGURE 5-1 Illustration of pain drawings from a 39-year-old woman who had experienced a whiplash injury 3 years previously. Currently, she reports pain in the neck region as well as in the jaws.

reported to influence quality of life, mood, and social relationships. When seen in the dental clinic years after a whiplash trauma, most patients will report that they think there was a tight relationship between the V pain and the cervical pain in terms of debut, development, and impact on function. Theoretically, there may be different options for a relationship (Fig. 5-2). In the attempt to dissect such difficult relationships, it may first be necessary to better define what is meant by V pain. In this chapter, we will focus primarily on the painful TMDs. The clinical classification of TMDs started with a landmark paper by

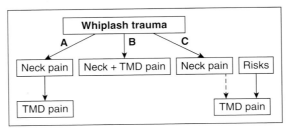

FIGURE 5-2 Theoretical relationships between a whiplash injury and neck pain and temporomandibular disorder (TMD) pain. **A** suggests a sequential relationship where neck pain "spreads" to the trigeminal region and may manifest as TMD pains. **B** suggests that the trauma is sufficient/adequate to directly cause neck pain and TMD pain. **C** incorporates the possibility that neck pain is only one of several risk factors for the development of TMD pain.

Dworkin and LeResche [7], who proposed a dual axes system with axis I being the physical presentation of the problem and axis II the psychosocial and distress part of the problem for the patient. Axis I was subdivided into (1) myofascial pain, (2) disk derangements in the temporomandibular joint (TMJ), and (3) pain in the TMJ and degenerative changes in the TMJ. It should be noted that not all TMDs per definition are painful (e.g., a clicking TMJ). The Research Diagnostic Criteria for TMD (RDC/TMD) has now been updated to the Diagnostic Criteria for TMD (DC/TMD), maintaining the dual axes approach but with validated and operationalized criteria for most of the painful TMDs [26]. A new entity termed Headache attributed to TMD has been added and serves as a link to the headache classification, that is, ICHD-3. In short, the DC/TMD allows an accurate and reproducible clinical phenotyping of the patients with V musculoskeletal pain.

Systematic reviews of the clinical overlaps between TMD pain and cervical pain related to a whiplash trauma demonstrate that a median of 35% of a TMD population will report a previous whiplash trauma that seems higher than the 2–13% in non-TMD control groups [11]. Furthermore, TMD patients with a history of whiplash trauma report more severe TMD symptoms such as difficulties in jaw opening, more intense TMD pain, and more headache and stress [11]. Thus, conclusions from such systematic reviews strongly support the notion that cervical pain and TMD pain are linked together and that the whiplash injury may be a significant risk factor, not only for the cervical pain, but also for the subsequent development of TMD pain. However, few prospective studies have been performed, and without valid information on the temporal relationship, it may be difficult or at least premature to draw very strong conclusions. One prospective study in a relatively small sample demonstrated that the incidence of TMD pain following a whiplash injury was no different from the incidence of TMD pain following an ankle distortion [15]. This is one of the few exceptions that used an active control group (ankle distortion) instead of a nonpainful control group, and the results from this particular study seem to suggest that whiplash injury is only a relatively minor risk factor for subsequent development of TMD pain. Obviously, this result needs to be reproduced in larger sample sizes. In the following paragraph, we will briefly review what is known about the basic mechanisms of TMD pain and sensitization.

BASIC OROFACIAL PAIN RESEARCH

Pioneers in the field of basic orofacial pain research have over the last forty years carefully and systematically examined the V nociceptive system and characterized the peripheral nocieptors, afferent fiber properties, V brainstem sensory nuclei, thalamic nuclei, and cortical networks [25, 27, 30, 33]. Key elements in much of this research are the convincing demonstration of the vulnerability of the V nociceptive system and the inherent property of neuroplasticity leading to peripheral sensitization and central sensitization and therefore changing the entire gain in the nociceptive system [4, 14, 34]. Moreover, pain modulatory systems—both inhibitory and facilitatory—have been shown to have a profound impact on the responsiveness of nociceptive cells and nocifensive behaviors in animals [22, 24] and humans [2, 35]. Recent research efforts have also emphasized the interplay between the V nociceptive system and glial cells [3] as well as the immune system [20]. In fact, there are strong indications of interactions between the nociceptive system and several other biological systems including, for example, motor function [10, 13], autonomic function [6], sleep [17], emotions [32], and cognitive function.

A sufficiently strong or unfortunate trauma to the neck and head could probably be the adequate stimulus to initiate the sensitization of the V nociceptive system, which then, by virtue of the neuroplastic changes and central sensitization, could maintain itself. In the following paragraph, we will address the structural and functional relationships between the V and the cervical systems as a basis for this V sensitization.

FUNCTIONAL AND STRUCTURAL RELATIONSHIPS BETWEEN V AND CERVICAL SYSTEMS

There are several lines of evidence to support the notion of an intimate relationship between the two systems in question. One is the obvious anatomical link between the head and the neck, and the simple observation that jaw movements are linked to head movements and vice versa [9, 12]. For example, maximum jaw opening is associated with a flexion of the neck. Second, there are strong neuroanatomical and physiological data with the extension of the caudal part of the V sensory nuclear complex into the cervical parts of the spinal cord as well as an extensive convergence between V afferent inputs and cervical afferent inputs onto nociceptive-specific and wide-dynamic-range neurons in the subnucleus caudalis [28]. Lesion studies with extraction of teeth in rats have demonstrated internalization of substance P receptors not only in the subnucleas caudalis but further caudal into the C2–C3 segment. Reflex studies in both animals and humans have also been seen as a support for the functional integration of the two systems; for example, stimulation of V afferent fibers causes short-latency reflex responses in the cervical musculature and vice versa stimulation of cervical dermatomes can also induce V reflex responses [1]. With the use of experimental pain models, it has also been described that moderate-to-intense masseter muscle pain can evoke changes in the electromyographic (EMG) activity of the cervical muscles and that experimental cervical pain can lead to changes in the V reflex sensitivity [16, 31]. Experimental masseter pain also influences the coordination between maximum jaw opening and the dorsal flexion of the neck. Interestingly, these experimental muscle pain models have shown that V muscle pain is rarely referred to the cervical structures, whereas experimental cervical pain is often referred to the V region [31]. Thus, there is ample evidence from different sources to support the structural and functional relationships between the V and cervical systems; however, it is still questionable that this may be the entire explanation for the spread of cervical pain to the V region. One reason to be cautious about overstating the importance of a whiplash injury for initiation and maintenance of V sensitization and pain is a series of studies that have identified not just a few, but a multitude of risk factors for TMD pain. These risk factors will be briefly described in the following paragraph.

RISK FACTORS FOR TMD PAIN

The Orofacial Pain: Prospective Evaluation and Risk Assessment (OPPERA)[1] study is a unique ongoing attempt to identify risk factors among several different domains, that is, clinical, autonomic, genetic,

---

[1] For specific details of OPPERA studies, the reader is advised to see original references.

somatosensory and psychological factors [29]. The use of the term "risk factor" in these studies is meant to reflect both etiologic events or experiences prior to the onset of TMD as well as contributory events or experiences that occur in parallel with the onset of TMD or exacerbation of TMD symptoms. An initial sample of 3263 healthy participants was carefully characterized with an impressive number of questionnaires, and clinical, somatosensory, autonomic, and genetic tests and techniques [29]. Subsequently, the participants were followed at regular intervals, and the number of new onset TMD cases was detected. From the analyses of baseline variables, estimates of risk factors expressed as odds ratios were determined. The outcome of the OPPERA study so far has outlined a wide range of risk factors that can be summarized thus: clinical risk factors—a total of 59 out of 71 variables demonstrated significant associations between baseline characteristics and new onset TMD pain patients, for example, history of trauma, parafunctional behaviors, and higher frequency of other pain conditions including headache [23]; several genetic risk factors, for example, COMT, serotonin receptor HTR2A, and more than 20 other SNPs (out of 3295 SNPs); autonomic risk factors, for example, heart rate; somatosensory risk factors, for example, pressure pain, mechanical pain, and heat pain (a total of 14 out of 39 variables); and, finally, psychological risk factors, for example, psychological and affective distress, stress and catastrophizing, and somatic awareness [29]. Furthermore, previous reviews have suggested that bruxism, occlusion, gender, widespread pain, joint hypermobility, and depression could be risk factors for TMD pain [5]. It seems clear from most recent studies that no single cause, event, or factor is strong enough to entirely explain TMD pain, and, therefore, a whiplash injury and cervical pain may be only part of the complex interaction between several mechanisms. In the next part of this chapter, we will present an approach that may serve as a new conceptual model for understanding the interaction between V and cervical pain.

STOCHASTIC VARIATION AS A MODEL FOR V PAIN

The basis for this approach to help explain complex biological systems comes from microbiology where bacteria with host-protective or virulent/damaging capacities would randomly interact to determine whether dental diseases such as gingivitis, periodontitis, or caries would develop or not as a consequence [19]. The principle of stochastic variation is also currently being discussed in various neurodegenerative diseases such as Alzheimer. In terms of V pain, given the assumption that there would be, for example, 100 meaningful factors per given individual to determine whether the person would become a V pain patient or not, there could be both risk factors (facilitating the development/maintenance of pain) and protective factors (inhibiting or counteracting the development/maintenance of pain), and each factor could have a different potency, varying from an arbitrary value of 0 (neutral) to 100 (extremely potent). If these factors just occurred randomly over a given period of time, then they would basically just be representing "noise" in the system. However, if there were interactions between the factors, and if they could have additive effects, then due to stochastic processes, there could be outcomes that would just oscillate in a nonpainful state, perhaps with some days better than others but never crossing an arbitrary threshold for symptom development and clinical manifestations of V pain (Fig. 5-3). If this mathematical exercise is repeated several times with exactly the same numbers (risk and preventive factors), different patterns or trajectories will emerge, and it becomes apparent that due to random variation, exactly the same risk and preventive factors may occur in a way that exceeds the threshold for symptom development and the pain condition could become "persistent," whereas in other cases (patients), the random interaction would generate only brief and transient types of pain. Fig. 5-3 illustrates some of the theoretical outcomes of such a simple stochastic processes.

The challenge in the stochastic variation model for V pain is, first of all, to determine the most important risk factors, and, secondly, to understand their relative potency and establish biological models supported by bioinformatics to determine the time course of interactions. This is obviously not an easy task, but the current proposal is intended to stimulate lateral and critical thinking in order to advance V pain research and as a plea to think in multivariate models rather than univariate models.

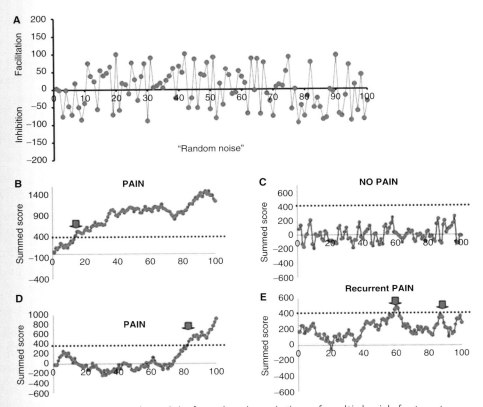

FIGURE 5-3 Proposed model of stochastic variation of multiple risk factors to explain different pain trajectories. The model assumes risk factors (facilitation) and preventive factors (inhibition) with potencies arbitrarily ranging from −100 to 100. If these factors occurred randomly with no interactions, an example of the outcome could be as shown in **(A)**. This represents basic noise levels, and no pain would develop. However, if there indeed were interactions with additive effects, then the outcome could be as shown in **(B)**. Here, due to the stochastic process, the risk and preventive factors (numbers) at the green arrow would exceed a theoretical threshold for symptom development (pain). Furthermore, due to the random effects, the summated "load" would remain at the "painful" level. At other occasions, the very same risk and preventive factors (numbers) would generate a completely different trajectory illustrated in **(C)**, and the summated "load" would never exceed the threshold for pain development. Yet again, if the same numbers are added but in another random sequence, pain may not be experienced before at a late stage (*green arrow*, **D**). The model will provide different trajectories and, as illustrated in **E**, may also account for recurrent pain conditions. Considering that a whiplash injury would be any of the risk (facilitatory) factors for development of TMD pain, it may be speculated that random effects could account for individual pain trajectories.

CLINICAL IMPLICATIONS

If clinicians treating V pain continue to think in univariate models, they would most probably address only one factor in the treatment plan. The controversy of malocclusion and TMD pain is a good example of univariate thinking with a straight-forward approach to the cure of the problem, that is, correction of the malocclusion by means of different techniques such as occlusal equilibration, occlusal rehabilitation, and orthodontics. For an updated review, the reader is referred to recent reviews in this field [21]. Nevertheless, based on the best epidemiological studies, malocclusion maintains to be a relatively low risk factor for TMD pain, and there must be a host of other risk factors at play (see OPPERA studies), and perhaps, whiplash trauma as discussed earlier. This scenario would call for other therapeutic approaches, and a suggestion could be that clinical benefit could be obtained from addressing cognitive-behavioral aspects of V pain [8]. There are a wide range of therapies in this domain, from simple information and counseling of the patients to hypnosis and mindfulness. Based on the stochastic model and the many different types of risk and preventive factors, and with due respect to the neurobiological mechanisms such as sensitization underlying most V pain conditions, it may be appropriate to also consider pharmacological interventions. The efficacy of most medications for alleviation of chronic TMD pain conditions has, nevertheless, been at least modest [18]. Numbers needed to treat values for most painful V conditions are typically in the range of 2–3 and the effect size around 30–40%. Perhaps with the exception of the triptans for alleviation of the acute migraine attacks, few true revolutions in V pain pharmacology have emerged. It seems that an approach combining cognitive-behavioral approaches, physiotherapy, and pharmacology would be a logical suggestion for most V pain conditions. With this in mind and if we can accurately phenotype and genotype V pain patients, then individualized and poly-target pain management would be a logical suggestion. As a final word, the intensity of the therapy may also vary during the time course due to the inherent dynamic nature of the interactions.

SUMMARY

This chapter has attempted to provide a short and unorthodox update on basic V pain mechanisms and a number of recently identified risk factors for development of TMD in relation to a whiplash trauma. A new stochastic model has been suggested to explain the possible interactions between not just a few, but many risk and protective factors at play. This model may help to understand individual time courses and pain trajectories. Finally, it has been suggested that univariate thinking in conceptual models and management approaches should be replaced by multivariate or poly-target approaches. There is a continued need for not only more but also better V pain research before we reach our ultimate goals of accurate and mechanistically based diagnostics followed by efficient and rational management of the individual V pain patient.

ACKNOWLEDGMENTS

Professors Ole Fejerskov and Firoze Manji are thanked for their inspiration of stochastical modelling in biological systems.

CONFLICT OF INTERESTS

The authors declare no conflict of interests.

REFERENCES

1. Bradnam L, Barry C. The role of the trigeminal sensory nuclear complex in the pathophysiology of craniocervical dystonia. J Neurosci 2013;33:18358–67.

2. Bushnell MC, Ceko M, Low LA. Cognitive and emotional control of pain and its disruption in chronic pain. Nat Rev Neurosci 2013;14:502–11.

3. Chiang CY, Dostrovsky JO, Iwata K, Sessle BJ. Role of glia in orofacial pain. Neuroscientist 2011;17:303–20.

4. Denk F, McMahon SB, Tracey I. Pain vulnerability: a neurobiological perspective. Nat Neurosci 2014;17:192–200.

5. Drangsholt M, LeResche L. Temporomandibular disorder pain. In: Crombie IK, Croft PR, Linton SJ, LeResche L, Von Korff M, editors. Epidemiology of pain. Seattle, WA: IASP Press; 1999. pp. 49–72.

6. Drummond PD. Sensory-autonomic interactions in health and disease. Handb Clin Neurol 2013;117:309–19.

7. Dworkin SF, LeResche L. Research diagnostic criteria for temporomandibular disorders: review, criteria, examinations and specifications, critique. J Craniomandib Disord 1992;6:301–55.

8. Dworkin SF, Turner JA, Wilson L, Massoth D, Whitney C, Huggins KH, Burgess J, Sommers E, Truelove E. Brief group cognitive-behavioral intervention for temporomandibular disorders. Pain 1994;59:175–87.

9. Eriksson PO, Haggman-Henrikson B, Nordh E, Zafar H. Co-ordinated mandibular and head-neck movements during rhythmic jaw activities in man. J Dent Res 2000;79:1378–84.

10. Graven-Nielsen T, Arendt-Nielsen L. Impact of clinical and experimental pain on muscle strength and activity. Curr Rheumatol Rep 2008;10:475–81.

11. Haggman-Henrikson B, List T, Westergren HT, Axelsson SH. Temporomandibular disorder pain after whiplash trauma: a systematic review. J Orofac Pain 2013;27:217–26.

12. Haggman-Henrikson B, Nordh E, Zafar H, Eriksson PO. Head immobilization can impair jaw function. J Dent Res 2006;85:1001–5.

13. Hodges PW, Smeets RJ. Interaction between pain, movement, and physical activity: short-term benefits, long-term consequences, and targets for treatment. Clin J Pain 2015;31:97–107.

14. Hucho T, Levine JD. Signaling pathways in sensitization: toward a nociceptor cell biology. Neuron 2007;55:365–76.

15. Kasch H, Hjorth T, Svensson P, Nyhuus L, Jensen TS. Temporomandibular disorders after whiplash injury: a controlled, prospective study. J Orofac Pain 2002;16:118–28.

16. La Touche R, Paris-Alemany A, Gil-Martínez A, Pardo-Montero J, Angulo-Díaz-Parreño S, Fernández-Carnero J. Masticatory sensory-motor changes after an experimental chewing test influenced by pain catastrophizing and neck-pain-related disability in patients with headache attributed to temporomandibular disorders. J Headache Pain 2015;16:1–14.

17. Lavigne G, Brousseau M, Kato T, Mayer P, Manzini C, Guitard F, Monplaisir J. Experimental pain perception remains equally active over all sleep stages. Pain 2004;110:646–55.

18. List T, Axelsson S, Leijon G. Pharmacologic interventions in the treatment of temporomandibular disorders, atypical facial pain, and burning mouth syndrome. A qualitative systematic review. J Orofac Pain 2003;17:301–10.

19. Manji F, Nagelkerke N. A stochastic model for periodontal breakdown. J Periodontal Res 1989;24:279–81.

20. Marchand F, Perretti M, McMahon SB. Role of the immune system in chronic pain. Nat Rev Neurosci 2005;6:521–32.

21. Michelotti A, Buonocore G, Manzo P, Pellegrino G, Farella M. Dental occlusion and posture: an overview. Prog Orthod 2011;12:53–8.

22. Millan MJ. Descending control of pain. Prog Neurobiol 2002;66:355–474.

23. Ohrbach R, Fillingim RB, Mulkey F, Gonzalez Y, Gordon S, Gremillion H, Lim PF, Ribeiro-Dasilva M, Greenspan JD, Knott C, et al. Clinical findings and pain symptoms as potential risk factors for chronic TMD: descriptive data and empirically identified domains from the OPPERA case-control study. J Pain 2011;12:T27–T45.

24. Ren K, Dubner R. Descending modulation in persistent pain: an update. Pain 2002;100:1–6.

25. Ren K, Dubner R. The role of trigeminal interpolaris-caudalis transition zone in persistent orofacial pain. Int Rev Neurobiol 2011;97:207–25.

26. Schiffman E, Ohrbach R, Truelove E, Look J, Anderson G, Goulet JP, List T, Svensson P, Gonzalez Y, Lobbezoo F, et al. Diagnostic Criteria for Temporomandibular Disorders (DC/TMD) for Clinical and Research Applications: recommendations of the International RDC/TMD Consortium Network and Orofacial Pain Special Interest Group. J Oral Facial Pain Headache 2014;28:6–27.

27. Sessle BJ. Acute and chronic craniofacial pain: brainstem mechanisms of nociceptive transmission and neuroplasticity, and their clinical correlates. Crit Rev Oral Biol Med 2000;11:57–91.

28. Sessle BJ, Hu JW, Amano N, Zhong G. Convergence of cutaneous, tooth pulp, visceral, neck and muscle afferents onto nociceptive and non-nociceptive neurones in trigeminal subnucleus caudalis (medullary dorsal horn) and its implications for referred pain. Pain 1986;27:219–35.

29. Slade GD, Fillingim RB, Sanders AE, Bair E, Greenspan JD, Ohrbach R, Dubner R, Diatchenko L, Smith SB, Knott C, Maixner W. Summary of findings from the OPPERA prospective cohort study of incidence of first-onset temporomandibular disorder: implications and future directions. J Pain 2013;14:T116–T124.

30. Stohler CS, Zubieta JK. Pain imaging in the emerging era of molecular medicine. Methods Mol Biol 2010;617:517–37.

31. Svensson P, Wang K, Sessle BJ, Arendt-Nielsen L. Associations between pain and neuromuscular activity in the human jaw and neck muscles. Pain 2004;109:225–32.

32. Tracey I, Mantyh PW. The cerebral signature for pain perception and its modulation. Neuron 2007;55:377–91.

33. Woda A. Pain in the trigeminal system: from orofacial nociception to neural network modeling. J Dent Res 2003;82:764–8.

34. Woolf CJ. Central sensitization: implications for the diagnosis and treatment of pain. Pain 2011;152:S2–S15.

35. Yarnitsky D, Granot M, Granovsky Y. Pain modulation profile and pain therapy: between pro- and antinociception. Pain 2014;155:663–5.

CHAPTER 6

Quantifying Dysfunction in Whiplash Injury
Old Questions, New Methods

James M. Elliott and David M. Walton

It is currently estimated that approximately 50% of people who report neck pain or related symptoms ("Whiplash-Associated Disorder," WAD) following a motor vehicle collision (MVC) will continue to experience persistent symptoms 12 months later [9, 91], with 20–25% experiencing significant long-term interference in daily activities [20, 73–75]. The signs and symptoms of persistent WAD vary from inconsistent to mystifying, running the gamut from localized neck tenderness or stiffness to cognitive and balance disorders with or without widespread sensory hyperalgesia [74, 76–78]. Despite the continued engineering advancements in the manufacturing of safer cars with improved seat designs aimed at preventing injury or death, the incidence of chronic or persistent WAD does not appear to be waning [81].

Adding to the complexity of the condition are inconsistent associations between subjective complaints and objective findings on traditional diagnostic imaging [15, 79]. Further, there has yet to be convincing empirical evidence that any form of active intervention is effective at improving the rates of recovery [36, 41, 50]. Several systematic reviews have concluded that the mechanisms of the event itself (e.g., direction of impact, speed of impact, awareness of collision) have little effect on the posttraumatic trajectory [88], while exaggerated negative affect appears to be one of the most consistent predictors of a poor outcome [7, 8]. The confluence of such findings has led to exploratory investigations centered on the key biopsychosocial factors that may drive the clinical course for some patients with WAD [17].

While the current literature in the field is offering promising new directions for understanding the etiology of this complex condition, much of it is being conducted in isolation or on one or few pathways, with few notable exceptions [38, 61, 83]. Although diverse, these advancements are offering potential points of interprofessional convergence that could be harnessed and applied practically toward knowledge transfer. This chapter presents an integrated perspective of WAD from biological, psychological, and social sciences that are intended to highlight potential points of convergence. By doing so, the intention is to highlight the complexities of the condition and propel whiplash research and treatment into a new era of understanding.

AN EVIDENCE-INFORMED INTEGRATED UNDERSTANDING OF PERSISTENT WAD

The broad spectrum of WAD signs and symptoms, including pain, sensory hypersensitivity, balance and neuromotor deficits [29], cognitive interference [3], and mood disorders [72], among others, suggests a multifactorial etiology. Foundational models to explain the genesis and maintenance of chronic posttraumatic pain (broadly) or WAD (specifically) range from purely cognitive [52] to purely biological [85], with recent attempts to integrate evidence from different fields [47]. A new adapted model is described in Fig. 6-1, describing the inciting event as a "trauma" that occurs within the premorbid biological (genetic, personal factors) and socio-environmental (medicolegal environment, support systems) context of the individual. Drawing from well-established models of stress and homeostasis [10, 42], the new model recognizes the experience of trauma and injury, whether physiological, psychological, or both, as a natural stressor to the organism that necessarily elicits activity in stress-response systems. The magnitude of the response is mediated by the magnitude or type of tissue injury, the genetic profile or physical habitus of the injured individual, peritraumatic emotional status, learned cognitions or coping strategies

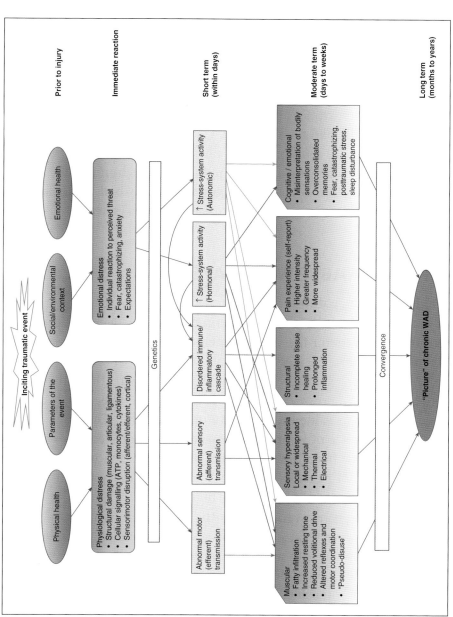

FIGURE 6-1 An illustrative depiction of a theoretical model describing potential interactions and pathways from the inciting event (trauma) to the picture of chronic Whiplash-Associated Disorder (WAD). Some pathways are established, others currently hypothetical but supported by emerging evidence

from a lifetime of experience, or even the responses from other important individuals such as family members, clinicians, attorneys, insurers, and others.

The terms are chosen intentionally to avoid judgment regarding the "correctness" of the stress response. Rather than choosing judgment labels such as "exaggerated" or "avoidant," the model describes such responses as adaptive or maladaptive, which demands consideration of the individual context; not all responses can be considered universally good or universally bad for all people. Consistent with previous models, two pathways are then proposed, one favorable and the other unfavorable. Even this may be an oversimplification, as human outcomes can rarely be dichotomized as clearly good or clearly bad, but it serves the purposes of this foundational discussion.

FAVORABLE PATHWAYS

To understand the pathway from trauma to recovery, it is prudent to first consider the outcome of, and definition for, recovery. There has yet to be consensus on the correct operationalization of recovery after traumatic injury. We feel a reasonable definition of recovery could include a satisfying end to the injury experience with the individual resuming, with little restriction, their preinjury life trajectory, including participation in valued roles and future goals [89]. This conceptualizes the experience of injury as necessitating a short-term deviation from life trajectory, but allows resolution of the dysfunction or, in some cases, redefinition or readjustment to a new satisfactory health status with or without medical/rehabilitative management.

We believe this is most likely to be the case when tissue damage is limited to contractile (e.g., muscle) or noncontractile (e.g., tendon or ligament) "soft tissue" with a stress response that is adaptive given the context. In this case, physiological or psychological processes, regardless of initial pain intensity, facilitate the restoration of relative allostasis (realignment with pretrauma status) through mobilization of key immune/inflammatory, endocrine, neural, and psychobehavioral resources, as will be described below. Notably, the sensorimotor system is largely spared in this pathway, in contrast to the unfavorable pathways described below. The coordinated adaptive efforts of stress-response pathways facilitate soft-tissue repair, encourage appropriate behavioral coping strategies, and provide a sound environment for a satisfactory outcome in a reasonable time frame.

UNFAVORABLE PATHWAYS

In this model, an unfavorable pathway can arise from damage affecting the peripheral and/or central nervous system (sensorimotor) in isolation from or in tandem with maladaptive stress- system activity. For purposes of clarity, these pathways are described as separate but parallel, although it is more likely that a bidirectional causal relationship exists between sensorimotor and stress dysregulation, where activity in one influences activity in the other. Accordingly, each will be described in turn.

Sensorimotor

Conceptually, the spinal cord is subject to the same mechanical forces as other spinal structures, yet it is one of the least elastic tissues in the region [16]. It is thus plausible that mild damage involving the ascending or descending white matter tracts of the cervical cord occurs during high-energy transfer of motion through the head and neck as occurs during MVC, leading to subclinical impairments in sensory and/or motor pathway signaling. Damage affecting the sensorimotor pathways may explain many of the signs and symptoms recently identified as part of the complex picture of chronic WAD, including thermal or mechanical local hyperalgesia [76] and widespread pain or hypersensitivity [67]. Damage to the motor pathways may represent a candidate lesion for explaining recent findings of muscle fatty infiltration in the neck (Figs. 6-2A, B and 6-3) [19–21, 23] or other muscles of subjects with chronic WAD (Fig. 6-4A–C) [22]. Such interference would also impair feed-forward activation (slowed time-to-activation) of the deep cervical flexors, which appears to be a consistent feature of chronic neck pain [27].

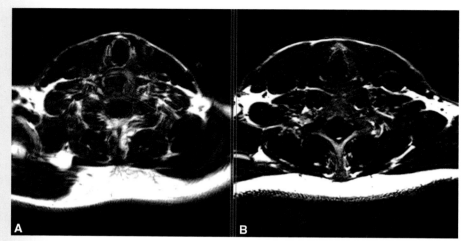

FIGURE 6-2 Axial (fat only) magnetic resonance imaging at the C6 level of **(A)** chronic whiplash and **(B)** recovered whiplash participants at 3 months postinjury. Muscle Fatty Infiltrates (bright signal) are clearly observed in the participant with chronic whiplash **(A)** but not the participant nominating full recovery **(B)**.

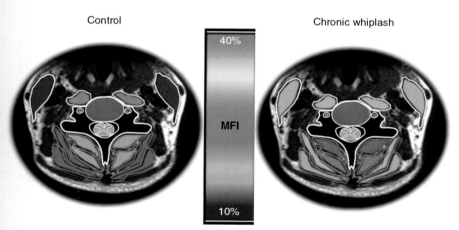

FIGURE 6-3 Heat maps detailing mean % muscle fatty infiltrates (MFI) in the extensor and flexor muscles from axial magnetic resonance imaging for healthy controls and chronic whiplash patients [19–21, 23, 25].

Preliminary evidence from our Chicago laboratory supports involvement of the cervical spinal cord in a subset of the population with severe chronic WAD symptoms [22]. Similar to other evidence involving patients with cervical myelopathy [34], spondylosis [65],

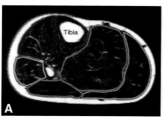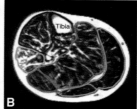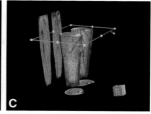

FIGURE 6-4 Axial (fat only) magnetic resonance imaging of the lower extremity musculature in **(A)** recovered and **(B)** chronic subject following whiplash injury, obtained from **(C)** 3D volumetric images [22].

and spinal cord injury [14], we have identified a subset of people with severe chronic symptoms that show signs of subclinical spinal cord damage using magnetic resonance spectroscopy [24] and magnetization transfer imaging (MT) [22]. Furthermore, using electric twitch interpolation techniques of the gastrocnemius–soleus complex, some subjects with severe chronic WAD demonstrated noticeable deficiencies in their ability to volitionally and maximally activate their plantar-flexor muscles, a metric referred to as the Central Activation Ratio (CAR) [22]. These preliminary observations of reduced CAR as determined with electrically elicited twitch interpolation, suggest signs of disrupted descending neural commands [5, 44] While preliminary, low CAR values in our participants (58–62% volitional activation) are consistent with previous results for quadriceps in those with known SCI [35]. Moreover, these reduced CARs have shown laterality preference related to the side opposite to which the head was turned at the time of impact, adding preliminary evidence for cause-and-effect. Supporting this, occupant postures of cervical rotation in addition to rapid hyperflexion/extension would appear to provide a prime environment for potential damage to various tissues [68] including regions of the cord that contain white matter motor pathways (Fig. 6-5A, B).

Preliminary (in preparation) work indicates that MT imaging could be used to identify changes in descending and ascending white matter pathways in the cervical spinal cord. Researchers in our Chicago laboratory used magnetization transfer ratios (MTRs) to measure the cervical spinal cord of 15 participants: five with moderate to severe symptoms (from 3 months to 3 years), five that self-nominated full

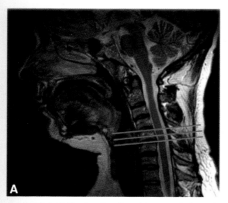
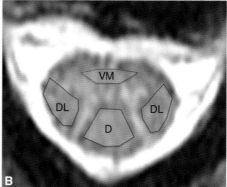

FIGURE 6-5 A: Sagittal T2-weighted MRI used to plan the **(B)** axial Magnetization Transfer Contrast image obtained using the Multiple-Echo Data Image Combination (MEDIC) sequence (with MT and without MT) used to calculate the MTRh. NB. Figure **(B)** is with MT pulse. (VM, Ventromedial; DL, Dorsolateral; D, Dorsal).

recovery at 3 months, and five healthy controls. The homogeneity in MTR response (MTRh), suggesting demyelination in descending white matter pathways, was calculated using region-of-interest analysis across the ventromedial, dorsolateral (left and right), and dorsal aspects of ascending and descending white matter tracts. The participants with chronic WAD had significantly different MTRh compared to healthy controls and recovered subjects ($P = 0.02$) (Fig. 6-6). In addition, MTRh was correlated with self-reported neck pain-related disability ($P < 0.01$) with the moderate/severe subjects having the largest MTRh values (WAD: 0.23, Recovered: 0.13, Control: 0.10) and higher mean percentage scores on the Neck Disability Index [84] (WAD: 44.4, Recovered: 1.2). Caution should be exercised until these results can be replicated in larger samples, and this work is well underway.

We and others have found that reduced PPT at anatomically distant sites (most commonly, the tibialis anterior) is related to poor, acute-stage prognosis [90], and may help identify an important subgroup of people in the chronic stage with global hyperalgesia [28, 80]. Furthermore, even when patients report unilaterally dominant neck symptoms, PPT measured over the most affected region and its contralateral analog have not shown consistent mean differences [90], requiring a

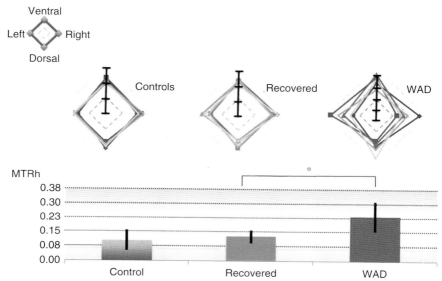

FIGURE 6-6 MTRh for the cervical spinal cord in 5 controls, 5 recovered, and 5 chronic WAD participants. *Asterisk* indicates significant group difference, $P = 0.02$.

reconceptualization of what is actually being measured with such quantitative sensory testing approaches (i.e., beyond an indication of local inflammatory processes).

We believe that global sensory hyperalgesia is another sign of central neurogenic dysfunction in these patients, further indicating impaired ascending/descending communication or cortical restructuring that are similar to other conditions such as Complex Regional Pain Syndrome [63] and chronic low back pain [31]. Pain thresholds and other such quantitative sensory tests (QSTs) are psychophysical measures, and it is logical to consider that those higher in trait stoicism in the face of pain are less likely to halt a pain threshold test early than are those more cognitively averse to pain. Our laboratory in London, Canada recently sought to address this commonly proposed cognitive mechanism of reduced PPT [87]. The results involving over 200 subjects with chronic WAD were largely not supportive of a strong cognitive component. Significant bivariate correlations were identified between local and distal PPT and pain catastrophizing, but not fear of pain, general depression, or general anxiety. After controlling for the effects of sex, age, and pain intensity, pain catastrophizing explained <6% of unique variance in PPT at either site, enough to be statistically significant but of questionable clinical relevance [87]. These results were also generally in keeping with earlier research in WAD [62] and in other chronic pain conditions [57]. While the mechanisms underlying widespread sensory hypersensitivity are far from clear, emerging evidence supporting interruption in ascending/descending pathways, while refuting a strong psychological component, are suggesting that *quantifiable biological processes* are strong candidates for explaining such phenomena. Disruption to ascending sensory spinal tracts, in particular, represents a prime candidate for explaining such findings. It remains plausible that evolving imaging applications could help to identify and objectify such changes [14, 22].

Stress-System Response

The human response to stress is distributed, complex, and highly coordinated. It is reasonably well established that both physiological [6, 12, 18] and emotional [40, 45, 70] resilience to stress appear to be at least partly under genetic control. The stress pathways represent attractive interactions between the psyche and soma, potentially offering biological explanations for the oft-cited relationship between early exaggerated cognitive distress and the persistence of post-WAD symptoms [82, 86]. While several stress-response pathways exist and continue to be found within humans, the most widely recognized hypothalamic–pituitary–adrenal (HPA) and broader sympathetic–adrenal–medullary (SAM) axes form the focus of this discussion.

The experience of trauma, whether physical or emotional, initiates a cascade of cellular processes and pathways that are intended to restore relative homeostasis of the organism. The SAM axis can most easily be considered two parallel axes: a neural cholinergic pathway, most represented by the locus ceruleus/norepinephrine (LC/NE) system that includes the autonomic nervous system, and the endocrine-based system termed the hypothalamic–pituitary–adrenal (HPA) axis. The cholinergic LC/NE pathway is characterized by increased sympathetic tone or reduced parasympathetic tone and release of adrenalin/noradrenalin onto target tissues in response to potential threat or stress [26, 56]. The HPA axis includes a cascade of neuroactive hormones that concludes with the release of the primary stress hormone cortisol: a glucocorticoid responsible for mobilizing key survival resources and for which receptors have been found on nearly every tissue in the body [11]. While their role is less clear, other neuroactive substances including Substance P and Ghrelin have also been implicated in the onset and maintenance of chronic stress conditions [49, 64], providing several potential biomarkers of distress that may partly explain the complex picture and outcomes of acute and chronic WAD and, germane to the previous section, known spinal cord injury [58]. A prolonged state of heightened physiological arousal (stress activity) has been associated with cognitive interference (impaired working memory or concentration), sleep disturbance, and widespread pain [11], all common in chronic WAD [69].

It has been demonstrated that HPA axis activity in response to stress influences the activity of pro- and antinociceptive cytokines [39, 46, 55]. Relationships have been shown between stress, serum or salivary cortisol, and concentrations of proinflammatory cytokines in otherwise healthy humans. Altered kinetics of IL-1α, IL-1β, and KGF-1 gene expression have also been shown in early wounds of restrained mice [48, 55], suggesting that prolonged or exaggerated cortisol release may interfere with the normal tissue healing cascade at the inflammatory stage of tissue repair, potentially predisposing the patient to chronicity. The second primary effect pertains to the connection between peri-traumatic distress and the formation of traumatic memories. Posttraumatic stress symptoms continue to be supported as risk factors for the onset and maintenance of chronic WAD [37]. Emerging research efforts attempt to explain the complex interaction between stress-induced glucocorticoid release and the development of fear-related memories by evaluating cortical neuronal signaling pathways such as the brain-derived neurotrophic factor (BDNF)/TrkB intracellular pathway [4, 30, 60]. Here again, a biological pathway is offering a link between early emotional distress and subsequent WAD-related signs and symptoms. As these fields continue to grow, new or modified pathways may be required to enhance our current understanding of the genesis of chronic WAD.

The "Secondary Outcomes" tier of the model attempts to provide explanatory convergence points for many of the clinical manifestations of this condition (Fig. 6-1). As described, impaired neurotrophic input resulting from disruption to descending spinal tracts coupled with prolonged, exaggerated, or blunted immune/inflammatory activity result in incomplete tissue repair, muscle fatty infiltration, muscular atrophy, and other signs consistent with disuse that have been termed "pseudo-disuse" out of recognition that these phenomena may be present even without any change in actual activity levels [25, 54]. Similar mechanisms, including nerve injury and inflammatory markers, have shown some relationship to sensory hypersensitivity in animal models [66, 92] and may offer an explanatory pathway for the same phenomena in chronic WAD. Cortical plastic change has been reported now in several chronic pain conditions [60], and WAD is not excluded [53]. At this point, the temporal development of such changes is unclear, but evidence is mounting that these may occur early in the postinjury trajectory [20] and are associated with long-term outcomes [1].

Cortisol has been implicated as a barrier to neuroplastic change, offering an enticing pathway for exploration in which acute distress leads to early cortical plasticity, which is then maintained through ongoing elevated cortisol. Impaired ascending/descending communication with the periphery, BDNF/TrkB signaling pathways [32], and even overconsolidated salient memories may all function as mechanistic explanations for cortical neuroplasticity that explain emerging findings from fMRI studies. Additionally, we believe the common clinical signs of cognitive interference, sleep, digestive, and widespread pain problems can at least partly be explained by prolonged physiological arousal resulting from ongoing stress-system activity. Finally, emotional interference, emotional detachment, or emotional lability are common in this condition [2, 13, 33] and may represent the clinical manifestations of prolonged arousal and memory over-consolidation. Collectively, these signs and symptoms converging at the picture of chronic WAD can potentially be traced back to sensorimotor system damage and maladaptive stress-system reactivity in the acute stage of injury.

DISCUSSION

This chapter has presented what we believe are potentially verifiable explanatory pathways to explain many of the diverse signs and symptoms often associated with persistent or chronic WAD. This has been driven by what anecdotally appears to be an increasingly pervasive skepticism directed toward those who develop chronic problems coupled with a paucity of empirically derived guidance for clinicians. Recent large randomized trials have revealed little to no effect of active intervention strategies for preventing the development of chronic problems [41], leading many policy makers to endorse a "wait and see" approach or a single session of advice and reassurance [51, 59]. We believe that better options exist, but before they can be properly explored, the mechanisms driving the clinical course of chronic WAD must be better understood.

This is not the first attempt to explain the genesis of chronic posttraumatic problems, and we are indebted to the pioneering work of those that have previously explored these issues [43, 47, 71]. To date, only the fear-avoidance model has enjoyed widespread adoption, but despite value for informing new cognitively based treatments for low back pain, it has not resulted in improved outcomes for WAD.

The intention of presenting a new model is to provide a "living" mechanistic framework that can be updated as new evidence becomes available, offering a platform upon which biology, psychology, and sociology can integrate to further understand this condition. While the stress-system aspect of this model has been proposed previously, this is the first time, as far as we are aware, that adequate evidence exists to propose a spinally mediated pathway that may hold relevance for exploring and developing more informed assessment and treatment decisions.

Naturally, there are caveats to this discussion growing largely out of what has necessarily been a selective review across a very broad scope of research fields. Readers should be aware that the model and brief discussion presented herein, while guided by existing and emerging evidence, is nonetheless prototypical and meant as a new starting point rather than an end point, and should be treated as such. At times, the emerging evidence has come from our own laboratories that has yet to undergo scrutiny through peer review, and so must be viewed cautiously. Where possible, works have been chosen that are considered seminal or particularly rigorous in the field, but no quality appraisals were conducted in keeping with the narrative purpose of this chapter. It is anticipated that with time and new research findings, some pathways will be modified, expanded, added, or removed.

In conclusion, this chapter has been developed in response to what appears to be an ongoing skepticism toward the patient with persistent WAD. Where traditional imaging has failed to identify a structural lesion, it is not uncommon that the chronic condition is considered to be multifactorial with both medical and noninjury factors influencing outcomes [17]. We do not disagree with this position, but our emerging interdisciplinary efforts suggest we can do better by identifying verifiable psychobiological pathways that show promise in explaining the seemingly disconnected spectrum of signs and symptoms of chronic WAD. While it is not exhaustive of all research in the field, it is intended to provide readers from a variety of backgrounds with a glimpse of the largely untapped potential for biopsychosocially integrated research to have an impact on a condition that is both common and costly and can lead to considerable suffering. The intention is to update this model on a 2-to-3-year cycle in order to keep the concept of WAD as a verifiable condition in the public eye.

ACKNOWLEDGMENTS

Funding for Elliott—Some of the work described was supported by the National Center for Research Resources (NCRR) and the National Center for Advancing Translational Sciences (NCATS), National Institutes of Health (NIH) through Grant Numbers KL2 RR025740, KL2TR000107, and NIH R01 HD079076-01A1 (NICHD/NCMRR).
Funding for Walton—Some of the work described was supported by the Canadian Institutes for Health Research and the Physiotherapy Foundation of Canada.

CONFLICT OF INTERESTS

Elliott has investment/ownership interest in a medical consulting start-up, Pain ID, LLC.

REFERENCES

1. Abbott R, Pedler A, Sterling M, Hides J, Murphey T, Hoggarth M, Elliott J. The geography of fatty infiltrates within the cervical multifidus and semispinalis cervicis in individuals with chronic whiplash-associated disorders. J Orthop Sports Phys Ther 2015;45(4):281–8.

2. Angst F, Gantenbein AR, Lehmann S, Gysi-Klaus F, Aeschlimann A, Michel BA, Hegemann F. Multidimensional associative factors for improvement in pain, function, and working capacity after rehabilitation of whiplash associated disorder: a prognostic, prospective outcome study. BMC Musculoskelet Disord 2014;15:130.

3. Antepohl W, Kiviloog L, Andersson J, Gerdle B. Cognitive impairment in patients with chronic whiplash-associated disorder—a matched control study. NeuroRehabilitation 2003;18(4):307–15.

4. Bennett MR, Lagopoulos J. Stress and trauma: BDNF control of dendritic-spine formation and regression. Prog Neurobiol 2014;112:80–99.

5. Bulow PM, Norregaard J, Mehlsen J, Danneskiold-Samsoe B. The twitch interpolation technique for study of fatigue of human quadriceps muscle. J Neurosci Methods 1995;62(1/2):103–9.

6. Burke SJ, Lu D, Sparer TE, Masi T, Goff MR, Karlstad MD, Collier JJ. NF-κB and STAT1 control CXCL1 and CXCL2 gene transcription. Am J Physiol Endocrinol Metab 2014;306(2):E131–E149.

7. Carroll LJ. Beliefs and expectations for recovery, coping, and depression in whiplash-associated disorders: lessening the transition to chronicity. Spine (Phila Pa 1976) 2011;36(25, Suppl):S250–S256.

8. Carroll LJ, Ferrari R, Cassidy JD, Cote P. Coping and recovery in whiplash-associated disorders: early use of passive coping strategies is associated with slower recovery of neck pain and pain-related disability. Clin J Pain 2014;30(1):1–8.

9. Carroll LJ, Hogg-Johnson S, van der Velde G, Haldeman S, Holm LW, Carragee EJ, Hurwitz EL, Côté P, Nordin M, Peloso PM, et al. Course and prognostic factors for neck pain in the general population: results of the Bone and Joint Decade 2000–2010 Task Force on neck pain and its associated disorders. Spine (Phila Pa 1976) 2008;33 (4, Suppl):S75–S82.

10. Chrousos GP. The glucocorticoid receptor gene, longevity, and the complex disorders of Western societies. Am J Med 2004;117:204–7.

11. Chrousos GP, Kino T. Glucocorticoid action networks and complex psychiatric and/or somatic disorders. Stress 2007;10:213–9.

12. Chrousos GP, Kino T. Glucocorticoid signaling in the cell. Expanding clinical implications to complex human behavioral and somatic disorders. Ann N Y Acad Sci 2009;1179:153–66.

13. Clementz G, Borsbo B, Norrbrink C. Burnout in patients with chronic whiplash-associated disorders. Int J Rehabil Res 2012;35(4):305–10.

14. Cohen-Adad J, El Mendili MM, Lehéricy S, Pradat PF, Blancho S, Rossignol S, Benali H. Demyelination and degeneration in the injured human spinal cord detected with diffusion and magnetization transfer MRI. Neuroimage 2011;55(3):1024–33.

15. Curatolo M, Bogduk N, Ivancic PC, McLean SA, Siegmund GP, Winkelsten B. The role of tissue damage in whiplash associated disorders: discussion paper 1. Spine (Phila Pa 1976) 2011;36(25, Suppl):S309–S315.

16. Czyz M, Scigala K, Bedzinski R, Jarmundowicz W. Finite element modelling of the cervical spinal cord injury—clinical assessment. Acta Bioeng Biomech 2012;14(4):23–29.

17. Dufton JA, Bruni SG, Kopec JA, Cassidy JD, Quon J. Delayed recovery in patients with whiplash-associated disorders. Injury 2012;43(7):1141–7.

18. Elenkov IJ, Iezzoni DG, Daly A, Harris AG, Chrousos GP. Cytokine dysregulation, inflammation and well-being. Neuroimmunomodulation 2005;12(5):255–69.

19. Elliott J, Jull G, Noteboom JT, Darnell R, Galloway G, Gibbon WW. Fatty infiltration in the cervical extensor muscles in persistent whiplash-associated disorders: a magnetic resonance imaging analysis. Spine (Phila Pa 1976) 2006;31(22):E847–E855.

20. Elliott J, Pedler A, Kenardy J, Galloway G, Jull G, Sterling M. The temporal development of fatty infiltrates in the neck muscles following whiplash injury: an association with pain and posttraumatic stress. PLoS One 2011;6(6):e21194.

21. Elliott JM, Courtney DM, Rademaker A, Pinto D, Sterling MM, Parrish TB. The rapid and progressive degeneration of the cervical multifidus in whiplash: a MRI study of fatty infiltration. Spine (Phila Pa 1976) 2015;40(12):E694–E700.

22. Elliott JM, Dewald JP, Hornby TG, Walton DM, Parrish TB. Mechanisms underlying chronic whiplash: contributions from an incomplete spinal cord injury? Pain Med 2014;15(11):1938–44.

23. Elliott JM, O'Leary S, Sterling M, Hendrikz J, Pedler A, Jull G. Magnetic resonance imaging findings of fatty infiltrate in the cervical flexors in chronic whiplash. Spine (Phila Pa 1976) 2010;35(9):948–54.

24. Elliott JM, Pedler AR, Cowin G, Sterling M, McMahon K. Spinal cord metabolism and muscle water diffusion in whiplash. Spinal Cord 2011;50:474–6.

25. Elliott JM, Pedler AR, Jull GA, Van Wyk L, Galloway GG, O'Leary SP. Differential changes in muscle composition exist in traumatic and non-traumatic neck pain. Spine (Phila Pa 1976) 2014;39(1):39–47.

26. Eskandari F, Sternberg EM. Neural-immune interactions in health and disease. Ann N Y Acad Sci 2002;966:20–27.

27. Falla D, Jull G, Hodges PW. Feedforward activity of the cervical flexor muscles during voluntary arm movements is delayed in chronic neck pain. Exp Brain Res 2004;157(1):43–48.

28. Farmer AD, Coen SJ, Kano M, Paine PA, Shwahdi M, Jafari J, Kishor J, Worthen SF, Rossiter HE, Kumari V, et al. Psychophysiological responses to pain identify reproducible human clusters. Pain 2013;154(11):2266–2276.

29. Field S, Treleaven J, Jull G. Standing balance: a comparison between idiopathic and whiplash-induced neck pain. Man Ther 2008;13(3):183–91.

30. Finsterwald C, Alberini CM. Stress and glucocorticoid receptor-dependent mechanisms in long-term memory: from adaptive responses to psychopathologies. Neurobiol Learn Mem 2014;112:17–29.

31. Flor H, Braun C, Elbert T, Birbaumer N. Extensive reorganization of primary somatosensory cortex in chronic back pain patients. Neurosci Lett 1997;224(1):5–8.

32. Galloway EM, Woo NH, Lu B. Persistent neural activity in the prefrontal cortex: a mechanism by which BDNF regulates working memory? Prog Brain Res 2008;169:251–66.

33. Gargan M, Bannister G, Main C, Hollis S. The behavioural response to whiplash injury. J Bone Joint Surg Br 1997;79(4):523–6.

34. Holly LT, Freitas B, McArthur DL, Salamon N. Proton magnetic resonance spectroscopy to evaluate spinal cord axonal injury in cervical spondylotic myelopathy. J Neurosurg Spine 2009;10(3):194–200.

35. Hornby TG, Lewek MD, Thompson CK, Heitz R. Repeated maximal volitional effort contractions in human spinal cord injury: initial torque increases and reduced fatigue. Neurorehabil Neural Repair 2009;23(9):928–38.

36. Jull G, Kenardy J, Hendrikz J, Cohen M, Sterling M. Management of acute whiplash: a randomized controlled trial of multidisciplinary stratified treatments. Pain 2013;154(9): 1798–1806.

37. Jull GA, Sterling M, Curatolo M, Carroll L, Hodges P. Toward lessening the rate of transition of acute whiplash to a chronic disorder. Spine (Phila Pa 1976) 2011;36 (25, Suppl):S173–S174.

38. Kasch H, Qerama E, Kongsted A, Bach FW, Bendix T, Jensen TS. The risk assessment score in acute whiplash injury predicts outcome and reflects biopsychosocial factors. Spine (Phila Pa 1976) 2011;36(25, Suppl):S263–S267.

39. Kiecolt-Glaser JK, Marucha PT, Malarkey WB, Mercado AM, Glaser R. Slowing of wound healing by psychological stress. Lancet 1995;346(8984):1194–6.

40. Kolassa IT, Ertl V, Eckart C, Glöckner F, Kolassa S, Papassotiropoulos A, de Quervain DJ, Elbert T. Association study of trauma load and SLC6A4 promoter polymorphism in posttraumatic stress disorder: evidence from survivors of the Rwandan genocide. J Clin Psychiatry 2010;71(5):543–7.

41. Lamb SE, Gates S, Williams MA, Williamson EM, Mt-Isa S, Withers EJ, Castelnuovo E, Smith J, Ashby D, Cooke MW, et al. Emergency department treatments and physiotherapy for acute whiplash: a pragmatic, two-step, randomised controlled trial. Lancet 2013;381(9866):546–56.

42. Lazarus RS, Folkman S. Stress, appraisal, and coping. New York, NY: Springer; 1984.

43. Leeuw M, Goossens ME, Linton SJ, Crombez G, Boersma K, Vlaeyen JW. The fear-avoidance model of musculoskeletal pain: current state of scientific evidence. J Behav Med 2007;30(1):77–94.

44. Lin KH, Chen YC, Luh JJ, Wang CH, Chang YJ. H-reflex, muscle voluntary activation level, and fatigue index of flexor carpi radialis in individuals with incomplete cervical cord injury. Neurorehabil Neural Repair 2012;26(1):68–75.

45. Loth E, Poline JB, Thyreau B, Jia T, Tao C, Lourdusamy A, Stacey D, Cattrell A, Desrivières S, Ruggeri B, et al. Oxytocin receptor genotype modulates ventral striatal activity to social cues and response to stressful life events. Biol Psychiatry 2014;76(5):367–76.

46. Marucha PT, Kiecolt-Glaser JK, Favagehi M. Mucosal wound healing is impaired by examination stress. Psychosom Med 1998;60:362–5.

47. McLean SA, Clauw DJ, Abelson JL, Liberzon I. The development of persistent pain and psychological morbidity after motor vehicle collision: integrating the potential role of stress response systems into a biopsychosocial model. Psychosom Med 2005;67(5):783–90.

48. Mercado AM, Padgett DA, Sheridan JF, Marucha PT. Altered kinetics of IL-1α, IL-1β, and KGF-1 gene expression in early wounds of restrained mice. Brain Behav Immun 2002;16(2):150–62.

49. Meyer RM, Burgos-Robles A, Liu E, Correia SS, Goosens KA. A ghrelin-growth hormone axis drives stress-induced vulnerability to enhanced fear. Mol Psychiatry 2014;19(12):1284–94.

50. Michaleff ZA, Maher CG, Lin CW, Rebbeck T, Jull G, Latimer J, Connelly L, Sterling M. Comprehensive physiotherapy exercise programme or advice for chronic whiplash (PROMISE): a pragmatic randomised controlled trial. Lancet 2014;384(9938):133–41.

51. Motor Accidents Authority. Guidelines for the management of acute whiplash-associated disorders—for health professionals. 3rd ed. Sydney: Motor Accidents Authority; 2014.

52. Nieto R, Miro J, Huguet A. The fear-avoidance model in whiplash injuries. Eur J Pain 2009;13(5):518–23.

53. Obermann M, Nebel K, Schumann C, Holle D, Gizewski ER, Maschke M, Goadsby PJ, Diener HC, Katsarava Z. Gray matter changes related to chronic posttraumatic headache. Neurology 2009;73(12):978–83.

54. O'Leary S, Jull G, Van Wyk L, Pedler A, Elliott J. Morphological changes in the cervical muscles of women with chronic whiplash can be modified with exercise—a pilot study. Muscle Nerve 2015; Epub Feb 20.

55. Padgett DA, Marucha PT, Sheridan JF. Restraint stress slows cutaneous wound healing in mice. Brain Behav Immun 1998;12(1):64–73.

56. Passatore M, Roatta S. Influence of sympathetic nervous system on sensorimotor function: whiplash associated disorders (WAD) as a model. Eur J Appl Physiol 2006;98(5):423–49.

57. Petzke F, Gracely RH, Park KM, Ambrose K, Clauw DJ. What do tender points measure? Influence of distress on 4 measures of tenderness. J Rheumatol 2003;30:567–74.

58. Previnaire JG, Soler JM, Leclercq V, Denys P. Severity of autonomic dysfunction in patients with complete spinal cord injury. Clin Auton Res 2012;22(1):9–15.

59. Financial Services Commission of Ontario. Minor injury guideline—superintendent's guideline No. 02/11. Canada; 2011.

60. Revest JM, Le Roux A, Roullot-Lacarriere V, Kaouane N, Vallée M, Kasanetz F, Rougé-Pont F, Tronche F, Desmedt A, Piazza PV. BDNF-TrkB signaling through Erk1/2 phosphorylation mediates the enhancement of fear memory induced by glucocorticoids. Mol Psychiatry 2014;19(9):1001–9.

61. Ritchie C, Hendrikz J, Kenardy J, Sterling M. Derivation of a clinical prediction rule to identify both chronic moderate/severe disability and full recovery following whiplash injury. Pain 2013;154(10):2198–2206.

62. Rivest K, Cote JN, Dumas JP, Sterling M, De Serres SJ. Relationships between pain thresholds, catastrophizing and gender in acute whiplash injury. Man Ther 2010;15:154–9.

63. Rommel O, Malin JP, Zenz M, Janig W. Quantitative sensory testing, neurophysiological and psychological examination in patients with complex regional pain syndrome and hemisensory deficits. Pain 2001;93(3):279–93.

64. Rosenkrantz AB, Mannelli L, Kim S, Babb JS. Gadolinium-enhanced liver magnetic resonance imaging using a 2-point Dixon fat-water separation technique: impact upon image quality and lesion detection. J Comput Assist Tomogr 2011;35(1):96–101.

65. Salamon N, Ellingson BM, Nagarajan R, Gebara N, Thomas A, Holly LT. Proton magnetic resonance spectroscopy of human cervical spondylosis at 3T. Spinal Cord 2013;51(7):558–63.

66. Schafer S, Berger JV, Deumens R, Goursaud S, Hanisch UK, Hermans E. Influence of intrathecal delivery of bone marrow-derived mesenchymal stem cells on spinal

inflammation and pain hypersensitivity in a rat model of peripheral nerve injury. J Neuroinflammation 2014;11(1):157.

67. Scott D, Jull G, Sterling M. Widespread sensory hypersensitivity is a feature of chronic whiplash-associated disorder but not chronic idiopathic neck pain. Clin J Pain 2005;21(2):175–81.

68. Shateri H, Cronin DS. Out-of-position rear impact tissue level investigation using detailed finite element neck model. Traffic Inj Prev 2015; Epub Feb 9.

69. Spitzer W, Skovron M, Salmi L, Cassidy JD, Duranceau J, Suissa S, Zeiss E. Scientific monograph of Quebec Task Force on whiplash associated disorders: redefining "whiplash" and its management. Spine 1995;20:1–73.

70. Stein MB, Campbell-Sills L, Gelernter J. Genetic variation in 5HTTLPR is associated with emotional resilience. Am J Med Genet B Neuropsychiatr Genet 2009;150(7):900–6.

71. Sterling M. A proposed new classification system for whiplash associated disorders—implications for assessment and management. Man Ther 2004;9(2):60–70.

72. Sterling M, Hendrikz J, Kenardy J. Compensation claim lodgement and health outcome developmental trajectories following whiplash injury: a prospective study. Pain 2010;150(1):22–28.

73. Sterling M, Hendrikz J, Kenardy J, Kristjansson E, Dumas JP, Niere K, Cote J, Deserres S, Rivest K, Jull G. Assessment and validation of prognostic models for poor functional recovery 12 months after whiplash injury: a multicentre inception cohort study. Pain 2012;153(8):1727–34.

74. Sterling M, Jull G, Kenardy J. Physical and psychological factors maintain long-term predictive capacity post-whiplash injury. Pain 2006;122(1/2):102–8.

75. Sterling M, Jull G, Vicenzio B, Kenardy J. Sensory hypersensitivity occurs soon after whiplash injury and is associated with poor recovery. Pain 2003;104:509–17.

76. Sterling M, Jull G, Vicenzio B, Kenardy J, Darnell R. Development of motor dysfunction following whiplash injury. Pain 2003;103:65–73.

77. Sterling M, Jull G, Vicenzino B, Kenardy J, Darnell R. Physical and psychological factors predict outcome following whiplash injury. Pain 2005;114(1/2):141–8.

78. Sterling M, Kenardy J, Jull G, Vicenzino B. The development of psychological changes following whiplash injury. Pain 2003;106:481–9.

79. Sterling M, McLean SA, Sullivan MJ, Elliott JM, Buitenhuis J, Kamper SJ. Potential processes involved in the initiation and maintenance of whiplash-associated disorders: discussion paper 3. Spine (Phila Pa 1976) 2011;36(25, Suppl):S322–S329.

80. Stone AM, Vicenzino B, Lim EC, Sterling M. Measures of central hyperexcitability in chronic whiplash associated disorder—a systematic review and meta-analysis. Man Ther 2013;18(2):111–7.

81. Styrke J, Stalnacke BM, Bylund PO, Sojka P, Bjornstig U. A 10-year incidence of acute whiplash injuries after road traffic crashes in a defined population in northern Sweden. PM R 2012;4(10):739–47.

82. Sullivan MJ, Adams H, Martel MO, Scott W, Wideman T. Catastrophizing and perceived injustice: risk factors for the transition to chronicity after whiplash injury. Spine (Phila Pa 1976) 2011;36(25, Suppl):S244–S249.

83. Ulirsch JC, Weaver MA, Bortsov AV, Soward AC, Swor RA, Peak DA, Jones JS, Rathlev NK, Lee DC, Domeier RM, et al. No man is an island: living in a disadvantaged neighborhood influences chronic pain development after motor vehicle collision. Pain 2014;155:2116–23.

84. Vernon H, Mior S. The neck disability index: a study of reliability and validity. J Manipulative Physiol Ther 1991;14:409–15.

85. Vetti N, Krakenes J, Eide GE, Rorvik J, Gilhus NE, Espeland A. Are MRI high-signal changes of alar and transverse ligaments in acute whiplash injury related to outcome? BMC Musculoskelet Disord 2010;11:260.

86. Walton DM, Carroll LJ, Kasch H, Sterling M, Verhagen AP, Macdermid JC, Gross A, Santaguida PL, Carlesso L; International Collaboration on Neck Pain. An overview of systematic reviews on prognostic factors in neck pain: results from the International Collaboration on Neck Pain (ICON) Project. Open Orthop J 2013;7:494–505.

87. Walton DM, Levesque L, Payne M, Schick J. Clinical pressure pain threshold testing in neck pain: comparing protocols, responsiveness, and association with psychological variables. Phys Ther 2014;94(6):827–37.

88. Walton DM, Macdermid JC, Giorgianni AA, Mascarenhas JC, West SC, Zammit CA. Risk factors for persistent problems following acute whiplash injury: update of a systematic review and meta-analysis. J Orthop Sports Phys Ther 2013;43(2):31–43.

89. Walton DM, Macdermid JC, Nielson W. Recovery from acute injury: clinical, methodological and philosophical considerations. Disabil Rehabil 2010;32(10):864–74.

90. Walton DM, Macdermid JC, Nielson W, Teasell RW, Reese H, Levesque L. Pressure pain threshold testing demonstrates predictive ability in people with acute whiplash. J Orthop Sports Phys Ther 2011;41(9):658–65.

91. Walton DM, Pretty J, MacDermid JC, Teasell RW. Risk factors for persistent problems following whiplash injury: results of a systematic review and meta-analysis. J Orthop Sports Phys Ther 2009;39(5):334–50.

92. Zhang J, Echeverry S, Lim TK, Lee SH, Shi XQ, Huang H. Can modulating inflammatory response be a good strategy to treat neuropathic pain? Curr Pharm Des 2015;21(7):831–9.

CHAPTER 7

What is Needed to Establish Valid Predictors of WAD Recovery?

Linda J. Carroll and Fatemeh Vakilian

WHAT IS NEEDED TO ESTABLISH VALID PREDICTORS OF WAD RECOVERY?

You are a clinician with a busy practice. You have in your office a 46-year-old woman who has neck pain after a recent car crash, in which the vehicle she was driving was struck from behind while she was waiting at a stop sign. The striking vehicle was going relatively slowly at the time of the crash, but could not stop in time due to icy conditions. Her current symptoms include neck pain and painful movement, with decreased range of motion and point tenderness, but no radicular symptoms. You know that your patient's prior health was fairly good, although in the past few years, she has had recurrent problems with mild depression. She is now anxious about driving, and is fearful about how long the neck pain will last. What can you tell her? Which of these factors and circumstances predict a shorter recovery course, which a longer recovery course, and which are unrelated to the course of recovery?

The ability to predict a likely health outcome is crucially important in clinical care and in health policy development. Identifying those factors that aid in accurate prediction (i.e., valid predictors) is a critically important form of research. There is a plethora of studies reporting predictors of recovery from whiplash-associated disorder (WAD); many of these studies contradict each other. The purpose of this chapter is to briefly outline some of the key questions to ask and aspects to look for when reading or conducting research whose goal is to identify valid predictors of WAD recovery outcomes.

WHAT IS THE STUDY DESIGN?

Predictors of WAD recovery can be identified only through longitudinal research in which the potential predictor clearly precedes the health outcome of interest. In cross-sectional studies (where all data are ascertained at the same point in time), it is generally difficult to be certain about temporality; that is, where the "predictor" and "outcome" are measured at the same time, it often cannot be clearly established which came first. An example of this is pain coping style and pain severity. A cross-sectional study may identify an association between these two constructs. But that design cannot determine whether a particular pain coping style leads to greater pain severity or whether greater pain severity leads one to be more likely to adopt that particular pain coping style. However, this is not the only danger in making inferences about predictors using cross-sectional findings. Take the example of a cross-sectional survey that finds a higher proportion of women than men reporting persistent pain after a traffic-related WAD. Temporality is not in question here: We understand that being female predates the injury. Indeed, these findings might indicate poorer neck pain recovery in women than in men. However, those same findings could instead reflect that women have a higher risk than men of having neck pain after a traffic crash. If that is the case, even if women and men experience neck pain recovery at the same rate, there would be more women with persistent neck pain in that cross-sectional sample, simply because there were more women than men with traffic-related neck pain in the first place. This is an example of prevalence–incidence bias, which arises because prevalence is determined by both incidence (probability that a condition will occur) and duration of that condition.

The longitudinal design most commonly seen in the WAD litera-ture on predictors of recovery is a cohort study. Ideally, potential par-ticipants are identified prospectively, enrolled in the study as soon as possible after experiencing a traffic injury, and are representative of the WAD population of interest. The study may compare recovery and predictors of recovery for different types of traffic injuries (e.g., WAD vs. ankle injuries) by following the cohort over time to assess similar-ities and differences in recovery of the two groups. Other times, there is no non-WAD comparison group, and all participants with WAD are followed over time to identify what pre- and postinjury factors predict recovery.

WHO WAS STUDIED?

The most valid predictors come from a study that includes either the entire population of interest (the "target" population), that is, a pop-ulation-based study that includes everyone with WAD in a particular jurisdiction or a representative sample of that population of interest. The target population—the population whom the researchers intend to draw conclusions about—should be clearly outlined in the study report and is defined by the inclusion/exclusion criteria. Representa-tiveness in the sample is crucial because otherwise you may introduce selection bias.

Selection bias is a matter of internal validity of a study, and can occur when the actual sample is different from the target population [10]. This can happen when, for example, only 50% of those eligible for en-rollment in a study (i.e., those meeting inclusion/exclusion criteria) agree to participate. Unless there is convincing evidence that respon-dents and nonrespondents are similar, it is likely that respondents are systematically different from those not participating (e.g., healthier or higher socioeconomic status), and this can lead to selection bias: the study findings may be incorrect. Selection bias can also be intro-duced through attrition. Dropping out from a study is rarely random, and a formerly representative sample may become nonrepresentative through, for example, selective attrition of those who are recovering very well or, alternatively, those who are recovering poorly. Where selection bias is present, findings are invalid unless the bias is taken into account in the analysis or the interpretation of findings. At the very least, there should be some attempt to compare participants with non-participants, and to compare those who complete follow-up with those who do not.

Generalizability is a matter of external validity [10]. Where there is low risk of selection bias (i.e., where the study sample is representative of the target population), study findings can be generalized to that target population as a whole. However, there can be no generalizability where internal validity is low. Note that a study that deliberately defines its target population narrowly but that obtains a representative sample of that narrow population does not suffer from selection bias. However, the narrow criteria that are used to define the target population will likely limit the researchers' (and readers') ability to generalize to a broader population; that is, such generalizations may not be valid.

WHERE DO STUDY PARTICIPANTS COME FROM?

In the current WAD literature on predictors of recovery, the most common sources of research participants are those making insurance claims for traffic injuries; those seen in ED after a collision; those enrolled/referred to intervention or other WAD studies, and "convenience" samples of persons recruited through newspapers, posters, etc. Each sampling frame has its strengths and weaknesses. For insurance sampling frames, some issues to consider when judging the likelihood of selection bias or poor generalizability to the broader WAD population are: Are there substantial barriers to seeking injury compensation? This will be highly jurisdiction dependent, since traffic insurance schemes vary widely. Can injured people obtain health care for WAD without making an insurance claim, i.e., does the claim's sampling frame "miss" many of these persons with WAD? Where there are multiple options of insurance carriers, are there patterns (e.g., different socioeconomic characteristics) of why people seek insurance from one company instead of another? To the extent that barriers to seeking insurance are minimal and most of those with WAD will make an insurance claim, where health care for traffic injuries is tied to making a claim and there is a single insurer for a particular jurisdiction, and where the study can ensure complete or almost complete inclusion of claimants in the study (or a representative sample), such studies reflect a representative sample of a target population of persons with traffic-related WAD. Thus, selection bias is minimized, and we can have more confidence that findings can be generalized to the larger WAD population.

Another sampling frame often utilized in studies of WAD recovery is using consecutive (consenting) persons seen at ED. However, the adequacy of this as a sampling frame is also jurisdiction dependent since patterns of going to ED after a traffic collision vary. In some jurisdictions, an ED sampling frame may miss up to 50% of those with WAD [7]. To the extent that those who go to EDs after traffic collisions are systematically different from those who do not (e.g., may be more seriously injured, more anxious about injuries, have better access to health care, and so on), this may introduce selection bias if the target population of interest was the broader population of persons with WAD. In addition, it is often the case that one particular hospital ED is selected for study, which leads to questions about whether there are systematic differences in those who go to that ED as opposed to another ED (e.g., those with more severe injuries may go to a particular hospital, socio-economic status may differ in those served by different hospitals, and so on). This, too, can introduce selection bias.

What about those sampling frames that include persons enrolled in intervention studies or referred to WAD research centers? The obvious advantage of this is that those agreeing to participate in intervention studies are generally more compliant, which will decrease nonparticipation and loss to follow-up and bias due to attrition. However, such participants may also be generally healthier and may be highly selected in other ways, so may not be representative of the larger WAD population to whom the researchers hope to generalize. In addition, when patients are referred to a study or a research center by their health care providers, we often have little clarity on how those health care providers made decisions about whom to refer and whom not to refer. Thus, not only may there be substantial risk of selection bias, but that bias cannot be well addressed in the analysis or interpretation of findings. Convenience sampling of volunteers recruited from newspapers, posters, and so on can be fast and inexpensive, but such samples are highly unlikely to be representative. Convenience sampling has an important role in pilot studies or in studies whose goals are generating hypotheses, but unless the researchers can provide clear evidence that the sample actually represents a target population of interest, these types of studies are also at high risk of selection bias.

Where sources of selection bias are known, they can often be adjusted for in the analysis [15]. For example, if the age distribution of participants and nonparticipants is different, a multivariable analysis can adjust for this. However, unknown sources of selection bias cannot be managed in this way, nor can the interpretation of findings take these into consideration very effectively.

WHAT INFORMATION IS GATHERED AND HOW?

Especially in the case of self-reported factors, such as postinjury pain intensity, it is usually best to measure potential predictors as early as possible after the injury. However, some potential predictors take some time to develop. For example, if pain coping style is considered to be a potential predictor of recovery in WAD, one must allow time for coping strategies to be tried and a pain coping style to develop. Neck disability is also a commonly used predictor. Yet, these questionnaires typically ask about how neck pain affects day-to-day activities. If disability is measured too soon after the injury, the individual will not have had the opportunity to assess how much his or her usual activities have been affected. In these cases, the potential predictor should be measured as soon as it is likely that such measurement will accurately reflect the construct of interest. If these measures are assessed too soon, participants' responses will not be accurate.

Similar to selection bias, information bias is also a matter of internal validity of a study [10]. Information bias can arise from errors in classification or in the measures used. This could include errors in the classification of persons with WAD as well as errors in classifying/measuring the predictor(s), the outcome and/or the confounders, and can lead to biased findings. However, unlike some forms of selection bias, information bias cannot be accounted for in the analysis. This highlights the need to ensure that studies use classification systems or measures with good validity.

Consider the example of a study in which prior (precollision) neck pain is the predictor of interest. We know from other research that when those with WAD are asked about prior pain, there is a strong tendency to minimize prior pain [3], which may be due to errors either in recall or in reporting. In the absence of other errors in measurements and if all study participants were equally likely to minimize prior pain to the same degree, this would lead to bias toward the null, that is, study findings are likely to underestimate any true association between prior neck pain and recovery. This is an example of poor sensitivity, that is, we are likely to misclassify those with prior neck pain as not having prior neck pain. Other measures have better sensitivity than they do specificity; for example, self-report measures of depression are more likely to classify people as depressed when they are not (low specificity) than to miss cases of depression. In general, the lower the sensitivity and/or specificity, the greater the likelihood that study findings will underestimate the true association [19].

Information bias may also arise when continuous data are categorized. In the WAD literature, recovery outcomes are frequently measures with continuous scores that have been categorized. Pain scores at outcome, for example, are often dichotomized into recovered or non-recovered. Disability scores are often categorized into no, mild, moderate, or severe disability. Although these cut-off scores have usually been validated, the sensitivity and specificity of the cut-off scores are never perfect, thus potentially introducing measurement bias.

Moreover, errors in classification of one variable are often related to such errors in another variable, as in the case of response sets where data are primarily self-report. A response set is the tendency of a person to have a pattern in how he/she responds, for example, to use the low end of a scale more than the high end or vice versa [16]. For example, a common outcome measure is neck pain intensity over the past week. If the person's response set is to endorse options on the low end of the scale, that will likely have been true for the baseline pain measures as well. Thus, the study findings are likely to show that low initial pain intensity is a strong predictor of better recovery, when in fact this effect may be due to response bias. This is especially a problem when the same instrument is being used to measure a predictor and an outcome (e.g., disability or pain measured at baseline and as an outcome) [16]. A more general example of this is "common method bias," where a common method (e.g., medical record review, interview, or questionnaire) is used to ascertain more than one variable in the study. This can lead to findings that either underestimate or overestimate the true association [15].

HOW ARE THE DATA ANALYZED?

Let us imagine that we have a study in which selection bias and information bias have been minimized. Does that assure that the identified predictors are valid? Not quite yet, because we need to consider issues related to the type of study, the data analysis, and presentation.

Evidence on predictors can be viewed using a framework described by Côté et al. [9], which classifies investigations into three phases. Phase I studies are hypothesis generating investigations, exploring, analyzing, and presenting the association between a potential predictor and an outcome in a descriptive, univariable way. Phase II studies are still exploratory, but explore, analyze, and present the role of a set of predictors. These studies present statistical models that include a set of factors predicting the outcome of interest. Although still exploratory, a convergence of results in a variety of samples and source populations increases one's confidence in the findings. However, caution is still warranted since correlations among sets of predictors can cause collinearity, which can lead to unstable statistical models, false positive results, false negative results, and/or apparent associations, which are in the opposite direction to the true association. Even where the associations among predictors are only moderate, such associations can lead to problems distinguishing the individual contributions of each covariate to the outcome [13, 17]. Phase III studies are considered confirmatory, rather than exploratory, and these are studies in which we can have the most confidence, although, of course, replication is always important. Phase III studies are large; have explicit a priori hypotheses; and examine the direction, strength, and independence of the association between a specific predictor and the outcome of interest, while explicitly controlling for confounding. A confounder is defined as an extraneous variable that is related to the predictor, a risk factor for the outcome apart from its association with the predictor, does not fall on the causal pathway between the predictor and the outcome, and accounts for all or part of the association between the predictor and the outcome [15].

To provide examples, the predictor "expectations for recovery" has been studied using all three phases of investigation. In a Phase I study by Vetti et al. [18], a univariable analysis showed that low baseline expectations for recovery (as the sole predictor in the model) increased the odds of poor recovery by 5.53 times. This sort of analysis is exploratory since it is possible that the effect of expectations could be explained away by a third variable (a confounder), but is very useful for generating hypotheses. More commonly seen in the literature on predictors of WAD recovery are Phase II studies. An example of such a study that included expectations of recovery as a possible predictor is from Bohman et al. [1], who assessed the role of a set of predictors: expectations, age, time between collision and baseline questionnaire, pain intensity, postcrash symptoms, prior pain, activity restrictions, health care utilization, and postcollision health. The multivariable analysis showed that expectations for recovery, age, days to report collision, pain intensity, and prior headaches were significantly associated with recovery. As an example of a confirmatory study on expectations for recovery, Carroll et al. identified a set of potential confounders (i.e., a variety of demographic and socioeconomic characteristics; prior health, injuries and pain problems; comorbid diseases; collision characteristics; postcollision symptoms, pain location, and intensity; and postcollision health care utilization). From these potential confounders, postcollision depressive symptoms, health, and neck and back pain intensity were found to meet the criteria for confounding [15]. After adjustment for these confounders, the rate of recovery of pain-related limitations for those with positive recovery expectations was three times higher than in those with poor expectations. Had this study not adjusted for confounding, the association would have looked much stronger, with an odds ratio of 4.5 [4], which is similar to that found by Vetti et al. [18] in their Phase I study. These three types of studies/analyses obviously answer slightly different research questions.

Especially when conducting multivariable analyses, having a large enough sample size for the analysis is also an important consideration. A rule of thumb is that for a dichotomous outcome (e.g., recovered vs. not recovered), there should be at least 10 events of recovery (or events of failure to recover) per predictor variable included in the model; for continuous outcomes, there should be at least 20 subjects per predictor variable entered into the model [11]. As an example, if a study of predictors of recovery versus failure to recover has 200 participants, of whom 50 have failed to recover, one should see a maximum of five predictor variables in the model to be confident that the findings are meaningful. A model that has too many predictors for the number of events may well be describing random "noise" rather than a genuine relationship.

SUMMARY

Valid predictors can be ascertained from longitudinal studies that minimize selection and information bias, and which have sufficient power for the analysis conducted. Where one is interested in the independent predictive role of a particular predictor (Phase III study), confounding should be considered; where the interest is in identifying a set of predictors, a Phase II study is appropriate.

To answer our clinician, the preponderance of low risk of bias evidence suggests that being female does not affect recovery (although it does appear to be a risk factor for WAD), and that older age is unassociated with pain recovery [5]. The evidence is still unclear about the role of prior health or whether those with WAD Grade II recover more slowly than those with Grade I (which may be because of misclassification bias) [5]. Collision-specific factors, such as being in the striking vehicle, do not appear to be predictive when other factors are also considered [5]. However, the preponderance of evidence suggests that the patient's postcollision anxiety and fearfulness do predict poorer recovery [2, 6, 8, 12, 14].

REFERENCES

1. Bohman T, Côté P, Boyle E, Cassidy JD, Carroll LJ, Skillgate E. Prognosis of patients with whiplash-associated disorders consulting physiotherapy: development of a predictive model for recovery. BMC Musculoskelet Disord 2012;13:264.

2. Buitenhuis J, Jaspers JPC, Fidler V. Can kinesiophobia predict the duration of neck symptoms in acute whiplash? Clin J Pain 2006;22:272–7.

3. Carragee EJ. Validity of self reported history on patients with back and neck pain after motor-vehicle accidents (MVA). Spine 2008;8(2):311–9.

4. Carroll LJ, Holm LW, Ferrari R, Ozegovic D, Cassidy JD. Recovery in whiplash-associated disorders: do you get what you expect? J Rheumatol 2009;36:1063–70.

5. Carroll LJ, Holm LW, Hogg-Johnson S, Côté P, Cassidy JD, Haldeman S, Nordin M, Hurwitz EL, Carragee EJ, van der Velde G, et al. Course and prognostic factors for neck pain in whiplash-associated disorders (WAD): results of the Bone and Joint Decade 2000–2010 Task Force on Neck Pain and Its Associated Disorders. Spine 2008;33(4, Suppl):S83–S92.

6. Carroll LJ, Liu Y, Holm LW, Cassidy JD, Côté P. Pain-related emotions in early stages of recovery in whiplash-associated disorders: their presence, intensity, and association with pain recovery. Psychosom Med 2011;73(8):708–15.

7. Cassidy JD, Carroll LJ, Côté P, Frank JW. Does multidisciplinary rehabilitation benefit whiplash recovery? Results of a population-based incidence cohort study. Spine 2007;32(1):126–31.

8. Cobo EP, Mesquida EP, Fanegas EP, Atanasio EM, Pastor MB, Pont CP, Prieto CM, Gómez GR, Cano LG. What factors have influence on persistence of neck pain after a whiplash? Spine 2010;35(9):E338–E343.

9. Côté P, Cassidy JD, Carroll LJ, Frank JW, Bombardier CH. A systematic review of the prognosis of acute whiplash and a new conceptual framework to synthesize the literature. Spine 2001;26:E445–E458.

10. Gordis L. Epidemiology. Philadelphia, PA: Elsevier; 2014.

11. Harrell FE Jr, Lee KL, Mark DB. Multivariable prognostic models: issues in developing models, evaluating assumptions and adequacy, and measuring and reducing errors. Stat Method Med Res 1996;15:361–87.

12. Kamper SJ, Maher CG, Menezes Costa Lda C, McAuley JH, Hush JM, Sterling M. Does fear of movement mediate the relationship between pain intensity and disability in patients following whiplash injury? A prospective longitudinal study. Pain 2012;153(1):113–9.

13. Pedhazur EJ. Multiple regression in behavioral research: explanation and prediction. Fort Worth, TX: Harcourt; 1997.

14. Pedler A, Sterling M. Assessing fear-avoidance beliefs in patients with whiplash-associated disorders: a comparison of 2 measures. Clin J Pain 2011;27(6):502–7.

15. Rothman KJ, Greenland S, Lash TL. Modern epidemiology, Vol. 3. Philadelphia, PA: Lippincott Williams & Wilkins; 2008.

16. Spector PE. Method variance as an artifact in self-reported affect and perceptions at work: myth or significant problem? J Appl Psychol 1987;72:438–43.

17. Tu YK, Kellett M, Clerehugh V, Gilthorpe MS. Problems of correlations between explanatory variables in multiple regression analyses in the dental literature. Br Dent J 2005;199(7):457–61.

18. Vetti N, Krakenes J, Ask T, Erdal KA, Torkildsen MD, Rørvik J, Gilhus NE, Espeland A. Follow-up MR imaging of the alar and transverse ligaments after whiplash injury: a prospective controlled study. Am J Neuroradiol 2011;32(10):1836–41.

19. Weiss NS, Koepsell TD. Epidemiologic methods. New York, NY: Oxford University Press; 2014.

CHAPTER 8

How Do We Prevent the Transition from Acute to Chronic Pain After Whiplash Injury?

Michele Sterling

Whiplash (WL) injury following a road traffic crash is common, with recent figures suggesting more than 300 persons (per 100,000 in the population) are seen in emergency departments every year in Europe and North America [7], and in Australia, WL injuries comprise ~75% of all survivable road traffic crash injuries [9]. Musculoskeletal conditions and injuries from road traffic crashes account for a large proportion of disease burden worldwide, with the burden associated with such conditions increasing [67]. WL injury incurs substantial economic costs, exceeding $350 million in Queensland, Australia from 2011 to 2012 [42]; in excess of £3 billion per year in the United Kingdom [31], and $230 billion US dollars per annum in 2000 in the United States [3].

Consistent international data indicate that approximately 50% of people who sustain a WL injury will not recover but will continue to report ongoing pain and disability 1 year after the injury [7]. Mental health outcomes are also poor, with the prevalence of psychiatric disorders in people with persistent whiplash-associated disorders (WAD) around 25% for posttraumatic stress disorder (PTSD) [40, 52], 31% for Major Depressive Episode and 20% for Generalized Anxiety

Disorder [36]. Individuals with poor mental health also report higher levels of disability and pain [14, 53].

In order to improve recovery rates and decrease costs associated with WL injury, it is important that clinical recovery pathways, mechanisms underlying the initiation and maintenance of the condition, and prognostic or risk factors for poor recovery are understood. Without this knowledge, there is limited basis on which to develop more effective treatments to prevent the transition to chronic pain. This chapter will first outline the above factors before discussing the implications for the development and testing of new treatments.

CLINICAL COURSE OF WAD AND PROGNOSTIC FACTORS FOR RECOVERY AND NONRECOVERY

Cohort studies have demonstrated that recovery, if it occurs, takes place within the first 2–3 months postinjury with a plateau of symptoms following this time point [34, 52]. Irrespective of long-term outcome, there is an initial decrease in symptoms to some extent in this early postinjury period. Two cohort studies (conducted in Denmark and Australia) have used trajectory-based modelling analyses to identify recovery pathways for disability, and both studies demonstrated similar results [2, 52]. The identified Australian pathways are illustrated in Fig. 8-1. These included: (1) a pathway of good recovery with initial mild to moderate levels of pain-related disability, and good recovery at 12 months with 45% of people predicted to follow this pathway; (2) a pathway of initial moderate to severe pain-related disability with some recovery but with disability levels remaining moderate at 12 months, with 39% of injured people predicted to follow this pathway; and (3) a pathway of initial severe pain-related disability and some recovery to moderate/severe disability, with 16% of individuals predicted to follow this pathway. The Australian study also explored mental health recovery pathways using the total symptom score of the Posttraumatic Stress Diagnostic Scale (PDS) [19]. Three very similar trajectories to disability were identified, and these are illustrated in Fig. 8-2—(1) Resilient: mild PTSD

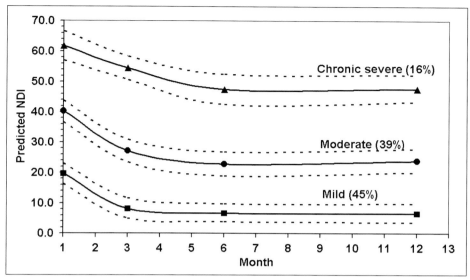

FIGURE 8-1 Predicted NDI trajectories with 95% confidence limits and predicted probability of membership (%). Figure reproduced from Sterling et al. [23], with permission International Association for the Study of Pain (IASP).

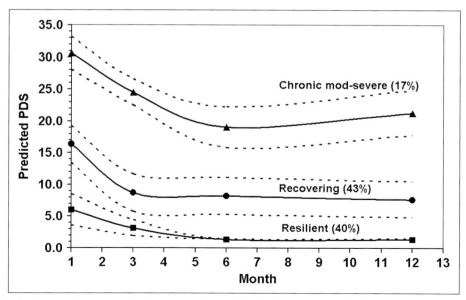

FIGURE 8-2 Predicted PDS trajectories with 95% confidence limits and predicted probability of membership (%). Figure reproduced from Sterling et al. [23], with permission International Association for the Study of Pain (IASP).

symptoms throughout; (2) Recovering: initial moderate symptoms declining to mild levels by 3 months; and (3) Chronic moderate to severe: persistent moderate/severe symptoms throughout the 12-month study period. Further analysis revealed a synchrony between the disability and PTSD symptoms trajectory groups, suggesting a common link between chronic WAD and PTSD development following WL injury [52].

The most consistent predictor of poor recovery following WL injury is the intensity of neck pain at the initial or baseline assessment, and this factor has been identified by all systematic reviews on this topic [10, 34, 46, 69, 70]. Walton et al. [69] synthesized the data from several cohort studies and established a cut-off point of 5.5 out of 10 on a visual analogue pain scale, with pain greater than this demonstrating a nearly sixfold increase in the risk of persistent pain or disability at follow-up. This factor was slightly more robust at predicting disability over pain outcomes [69]. Initial moderate-to-high levels of pain-related disability have also shown predictive capacity [57]. Interestingly, this is also the case for chronic pain development postsurgery and serious trauma. Higher levels of pain either before or in the acute postsurgery period are associated with an increased risk of developing chronic pain [1, 21, 24]. Initial pain severity has also been shown to predict chronic pain 12 months after serious orthopedic injury [27].

Mechanisms underlying higher levels of reported pain are not clear, but their elucidation may provide potential targets for treatment. Several studies have investigated the prognostic capacity of sensory measures with the aim of providing information on potential nociceptive processes that may underlie the development of chronic WL pain. Cold hyperalgesia predicted disability and mental health outcomes at 12 months postinjury [53, 55], and decreased cold pain tolerance measured with the cold pressor test predicted ongoing disability [35]. A recent systematic review concluded that there is now moderate evidence available to support cold hyperalgesia as an adverse prognostic indicator [22]. Other sensory measures such as lowered pressure pain thresholds (mechanical hyperalgesia) show inconsistent prognostic capacity. Walton et al. [68] showed that decreased pressure pain thresholds over a distal site in the leg predicted neck pain-related disability at 3 months postinjury, but other studies have shown that this factor is not an independent predictor of later disability [55]. The exact mechanisms underlying the hyperalgesic responses are not clearly understood, but are generally acknowledged to reflect augmented nociceptive processing in the central nervous system (central sensitization or less of descending inhibition) [11, 58].

Psychological factors that have shown the most consistent prognostic capacity for WAD outcomes include posttraumatic stress symptoms, pain catastrophizing, and symptoms of depressed mood [7, 54, 69]. Additionally, lower expectations of recovery have been shown to predict poor recovery where patients who do not expect to recover well may not do so [6, 26].

Most prognostic studies of WAD have been Phase 1 or exploratory studies with few confirmatory or validation studies yet conducted [50]. A recent study undertook validation of a set of prognostic indicators including initial disability, cold hyperalgesia, age, and posttraumatic stress symptoms. The results indicated that the predictive set showed good accuracy to discriminate patients with moderate/severe disability from patients with full recovery or residual milder symptoms at 12 months postinjury [54]. Such a validation study is rare in this area of research and goes some way toward providing greater confidence for the use of these measures in the early assessment of WL injury.

On the basis of results of previous cohort studies, a clinical prediction rule to identify both chronic moderate/severe disability and full recovery at 12 months postinjury was recently developed [44, 45]. The aim of the rule is to provide clinicians with a useful screening tool to gauge the risk of an individual patient developing a chronic condition. Initial disability levels (Neck Disability Index [NDI] score of ≥40%), age ≥35 years, and a score of ≥6 on the hyperarousal subscale of the PDS [20] could predict patients with moderate/severe disability at 12 months with good specificity, fair sensitivity, and a positive predictive value of 72% [45]. It is also important to predict patients who will recover well as these patients will likely require less intensive intervention. Initial NDI scores of ≤32% and age ≤35 years predicted full recovery at 12 months postinjury with a positive predictive value of 71% [45]. A third medium risk group could either recover or develop chronic pain and disability (>32% on the NDI, score >3 on

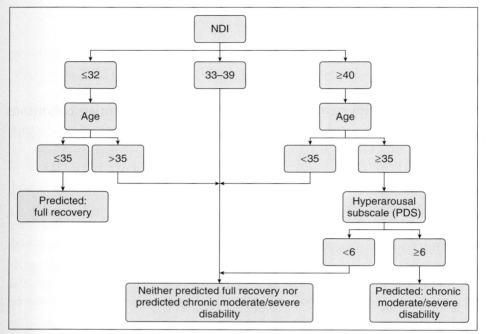

FIGURE 8-3 Whiplash CPR [46] to predict both chronic moderate/severe disability and full recovery following an acute whiplash injury. (Reprinted with permission from Ritchie et al. [45].)

the hyperarousal subscale). The hyperarousal subscale comprises 5 items that evaluate the frequency of symptoms including: having trouble falling asleep, feelings of irritability, difficulty concentrating, being overly alert, and being easily startled. The clinical prediction rule has subsequently been externally validated in an independent cohort and the reproducibility and accuracy of this dual pathway tool have been confirmed for individuals with acute WAD [44]. It is illustrated in Fig. 8-3.

ETIOLOGICAL PROCESSES IN WAD

Although controversial, there is converging evidence available indicating the presence of a peripheral lesion in some individuals after WL injury [12] and that such lesions may persist beyond what is considered the usual time for healing of soft tissues [48]. There is also evidence that a lesion may not be a prerequisite for some of the clinical features of patients with WAD. For example, pain and hyperalgesia can be present in individuals with stress-related conditions but without a specific injury [13]. Additionally, in most injured people, a lesion cannot be established with current imaging technology, and in other conditions even if lesions or pathology are present, they do not correlate well with levels of pain and disability [65]. For these reasons, it is important to consider processes that may underlie the initiation of WL pain and maintenance of symptoms in those who do not recover as this may provide opportunity for the development of more effective interventions targeted toward these processes.

There are clear movement- and motor-related disturbances in patients with acute and chronic WAD. A loss of range of neck movement is a cardinal sign that forms the basis of the classification system of the condition [49]. Changes also include altered muscle recruitment patterns [56], morphological changes in neck muscles [17], disturbed eye movement control, loss of balance, and joint repositioning errors [64], with most of these changes being identified in both acute and chronic WAD. Although the majority of these movement/motor changes are seen in all neck pain regardless of onset, greater dysfunction appears to be more apparent in WAD (traumatic-onset neck pain). For example, the presence of fatty infiltrate in the cervical flexors and extensors, clearly present in WAD but not in nontraumatic onset neck pain [15, 16]. The cause of the fatty infiltrate and its implications for treatment are not clear.

Additionally, it seems that the sensory presentation of traumatic and nontraumatic neck pain is different, with the inference being that nociceptive processing is different between the two forms of neck pain. Two recent systematic reviews have concluded that there is moderate evidence that the sensory presentation of widespread sensory hypersensitivity at sites both local and remote to the injured area found in chronic WAD indicates the presence of augmented nociceptive processing or sensitization within the central nervous system [58, 66]. Later findings would support this with clear evidence of spinal cord hyperexcitability [39] as well as impaired descending inhibitory mechanisms [43]. While there are some reports of similar findings indicative of central sensitization in nontraumatic neck pain when compared to healthy controls [30], direct comparisons of nontraumatic neck pain and WAD have shown more pronounced sensory disturbances in the latter traumatic neck pain group [8, 15, 47]. These findings suggest different nociceptive processing mechanisms may underlie neck pain, depending on whether or not it is of traumatic onset, and this could be one reason for apparently better responses to physical treatments in patients with nontraumatic neck pain [33, 41].

As with any painful musculoskeletal condition, relationships between psychological factors and health outcomes have been well documented, and this is no different for WL. It is generally considered that psychological factors alone do not fully explain poor recovery following the injury but that they likely interact with other processes and play a role in the persistence of symptoms (see chapter by Turk and Robinson in this volume). Psychological factors may be pain related such as fear of movement due to pain [5] and pain catastrophizing [60], among others. Psychological factors related to the injury event itself also play a role. PTSD is common psychological sequelae following a road traffic crash [37], and there is increasing recognition of a shared pattern of etiology between WAD and PTSD [29]. Recent data indicate that PTSD symptoms are prevalent in individuals who have sustained WL injuries following a road traffic crash [4, 61] and up to 25% of those with chronic WAD have a diagnosis of probable PTSD [52]. The early presence of posttraumatic stress symptoms has been shown to be associated with poor functional recovery from the injury [4, 54].

Additionally, psychological distress related to environmental and social factors may also be involved. Perceived injustice in relation to pain is defined as an appraisal reflecting the severity and irreparability of pain-related loss, blame, and unfairness [61], and has been shown to predict prolonged work absence after WL injury [59]. A later study demonstrated that perceived injustice predicted ongoing symptoms of posttraumatic stress [61]. Additionally, stress associated with compensation claim lodgment may also influence recovery following injury, with a recent study showing that reported stress around medicolegal assessment, claim delays, and understanding claims predicted ongoing disability and poorer quality of life [23].

Individuals with WAD often report a diverse range of symptoms including dizziness, nausea, upper and lower limb paresthesia, tinnitus, cognitive difficulties, and generalized sensory disturbances, and this has led to proposals that it is a systemic type of general illness rather than an isolated neck pain condition [18]. Recent findings of elevated serum levels of the inflammatory biomarker, C-reactive protein, in that acute stage of injury that persisted in those who developed a chronic condition provide support for this tenet [51]. C-reactive protein levels showed moderate correlations with mechanical hyperalgesia both locally over the cervical spine and at a remote lower limb location as well as with thermal (heat and cold) hyperalgesia, indicating that low-level systemic inflammation may also play a role in the presentation of WAD [51].

It is apparent that numerous and varied but interrelating processes are likely involved in the initiation and maintenance of WAD symptoms (see also Turk and Robinson chapter in this volume). It is not clear which processes are causally related to health outcomes and which are epiphenomena associated with the condition. Nevertheless, some of these processes offer potential as targets for future treatments, and these will be discussed below.

THE TREATMENT OF ACUTE WAD

The treatment of WAD in the acute/subacute stage of the injury (up to 12 weeks) will be important to achieve the goal of reducing the numbers of injured people who develop chronic pain. The most recent systematic reviews conclude that activity- and/or exercise-based interventions are the most effective conservative treatments for acute WAD but that effects are modest and the relative effectiveness of various exercise regimes is not clear [62, 63].

Two additional randomized controlled trials have been conducted since these reviews, again demonstrating only modest effects. One conducted in emergency departments of UK hospitals demonstrated that six sessions of physiotherapy (a multimodal approach of exercise, manual therapy) were only slightly more effective, but not more cost effective, than a single session of advice from a physiotherapist [38]. Only 45–50% of participants in either treatment group reported their condition as being "much better" or "better" at short- (4 months) and long-term follow-up (12 months)—a low recovery rate that is little different than the usual natural recovery following the injury [52]. Another recent randomized controlled trial investigated whether the early targeting of processes including motor dysfunction, central sensitization, and psychological distress would provide better outcomes than usual care [32]. Participants with acute WAD (≤4 weeks duration) were assessed using measures of pain, disability, sensory function, and psychological questionnaires including general distress and posttraumatic stress symptoms. Treatment was tailored to the findings of the assessment and could range from a physiotherapy program of advice, exercise, and manual therapy for those with few signs of central hyperexcitability and psychological distress to an interdisciplinary intervention comprising medication (for greater than moderate pain and signs of central sensitization) and cognitive-behavioral therapy delivered by a clinical psychologist (if scores on psychological questionnaires were above threshold). This pragmatic intervention approach was compared to usual care where the patient received treatment as they normally would. There were no significant differences in frequency of recovery (defined as NDI <8%) between the two intervention groups at 6 or 12 months, demonstrating no benefit of the early interdisciplinary intervention [32]. Several possible reasons for these results were proposed. The design of the trial may have been too broad and not sensitive enough to detect changes in subgroups of patients, suggesting better outcomes would be achieved by specifically selecting patients at high risk of poor recovery. Additionally, 61% of participants in the trial found the medication (low-dose opioids and/or adjuvant agents) to be unacceptable due to side effects such as dizziness and drowsiness, and did not comply with the prescribed dose, [32], indicating that more acceptable medications need to be evaluated. Compliance with attending sessions with the clinical psychologist was less than that with physiotherapy, perhaps indicating patient preference for physiotherapy.

The results of the above-mentioned trial should not negate attempts to address and target potentially modifiable risk factors in the early injury stage. There were, as outlined, several methodological issues that may have influenced the results. Risk factors (prognostic indicators) for chronic pain development following WL injury are not necessarily causal factors, but targeting these processes in a systematic way would seem a logical approach to move this field forward. Such an approach has been explored in the area of low back pain, where stratified care was provided to patients, depending upon their risk of developing chronic pain and disability, with results showing some promise [25]. As outlined earlier, we recently developed and validated a clinical prediction rule that identifies patients at high and low risk of poor and good recovery with good specificity and adequate sensitivity [44, 45]. Whether or not the use of a stratified pathway of care for WL can improve recovery remains to be seen.

Patients identified as being at low risk of poor recovery will likely require less intensive treatment that, intuitively, could comprise advice, assurance, together with simple exercises, but this proposal requires formal testing. Patients at medium or high risk for poor recovery will likely need additional treatments to the basic advice/activity/exercise approach. This may include strategies to target pain and nociceptive processes as well as methods to address early psychological responses to injury. As can be seen in a recent trial by Jull et al. [32], this approach may not be straightforward. The participants in this trial not only found the side effects of medication unacceptable but also were less compliant with attendance to a clinical psychologist (46% of participants attended fewer than 4 of 10 sessions) compared to attendance with the physiotherapist (12% attended fewer than 4 sessions over 10 weeks) [32]. The reasons for noncompliance are not clear, but the burden of attending numerous health care visits with different practitioners may have played a role. An alternative approach, currently being evaluated, is to train physiotherapists to deliver psychological interventions and to play a more "gatekeeper" role in the early assessment, risk stratification, and triaging of patients with acute WAD. This approach has been investigated in mainly chronic conditions such as arthritis [28] as well as in acute low back pain [25], and results have shown some early promise. This is not to say that patients with a diagnosed psychopathology such as depression or PTSD should be managed by physiotherapists, and these patients will require referral to an appropriately trained professional.

CONCLUSION

We are at the crossroads in the research and clinical management of acute and chronic WAD. The evidence is demonstrating that the recommended treatment approaches that comprise predominantly of activity or exercise provide only small effects. This is not to say that exercise-based interventions should not be provided to people with WAD, as exercise and activity are important for long-term general health. It may be that activity/exercise is combined with other treatments that target consistently identified risk factors such as aberrant nociceptive processing, psychological factors, stress, and immune processes, as well as improving system and environmental factors to minimize psychological distress. The relationships between risk factors and their development and causal relationship to outcomes as well as the testing of new interventions would seem a logical progression of research in this area.

ACKNOWLEDGMENT

MS receives a Fellowship from the National Health and Medical Research Council, Australia.

REFERENCES

1. Aasvang E, Gmaehle E, Hansen JB, Gmaehle B, Forman JL, Schwarz J, Bittner R, Kehlet H. Predictive risk factors for persistent postherniotomy pain. Anesthesiology 2010;112(4):957–69.

2. Andersen T, Karstoft K, Brink O, Elklit A. Trajectories of pain symptoms following whiplash injury: a prospective cohort study. Proceedings of the 8th Congress of the European Pain Federation EFIC. Florence: EFIC; 2013. p. 39.

3. Blincoe L, Seay A, Zaloshnja E, Miller T, Romano E, Luchter S, Spicer R. The economic impact of motor vehicle crashes, 2000 (DOT HS 809 446). Washington, DC: National Highway Traffic Safety Administration; 2002.

4. Buitenhuis J, DeJong J, Jaspers J, Groothoff J. Relationship between posttraumatic stress disorder symptoms and the course of whiplash complaints. J Psychosom Res 2006;61(3):681–9.

5. Buitenhuis J, Jaspers J, Fidler V. Can kinesiophobia predict the duration of neck symptoms in acute whiplash? Clin J Pain 2006;22(3):272–7.

6. Carroll L, Holm L, Ferrari R, Ozegovic D, Cassidy D. Recovery in whiplash-associated disorders: do you get what you expect. J Rheumatol 2009;36:1063–70.

7. Carroll LJ, Holm LW, Hogg-Johnson S, Côté P, Cassidy JD, Haldeman S, Nordin M, Hurwitz EL, Carragee EJ, van der Velde G, et al. Course and prognostic factors for neck pain in whiplash-associated disorders (WAD): results of the Bone and Joint Decade 2000–2010 Task Force on Neck Pain and Its Associated Disorders. Spine (Phila Pa 1976) 2008;33(4, Suppl):S83–S92.

8. Chien A, Eliav E, Sterling M. Sensory hypoaesthesia is a feature of chronic whiplash but not chronic idiopathic neck pain. Manual Therapy 2010;15(1):48–53.

9. Connelly L, Supangan R. The economic costs of road traffic crashes: Australia, states and territories. Accid Anal Prev 2006;38:1087–93.

10. Cote P, Cassidy D, Carroll L, Frank J, Bombardier C. A systematic review of the prognosis of acute whiplash and a new conceptual framework to synthesize the literature. Spine 2001;26(19):E445–E458.

11. Curatolo M, Arendt-Nielsen L, Petersen-Felix S. Evidence, mechanisms and clinical implications of central hypersensitivity in chronic pain after whiplash injury. Clin J Pain 2004;20(6):469–76.

12. Curatolo M, Bogduk N, Ivancic P, McLean S, Siegmund G, Winkelstein B. The role of tissue damage in whiplash associated disorders. Spine 2011;36(25, Suppl):S309–S315.

13. Defrin R, Ginzburg K, Solomon Z, Polad E, Bloch M, Govezensky M, Schreiber S. Quantitative testing of pain perception in subjects with PTSD—implications for the mechanism of the coexistence between PTSD and chronic pain. Pain 2008;138(2):450–9.

14. Dunne R, Kenardy J, Sterling M. A randomised controlled trial of cognitive behavioural therapy for the treatment of PTSD in the context of chronic whiplash. Clin J Pain 2012;28(9):755–65.

15. Elliott J, Jull G, Sterling M, Noteboom T, Darnell R, Galloway G. Fatty infiltrate in the cervical extensor muscles is not a feature of chronic insidious onset neck pain. Clin Radiol 2008;63(6):681–7.

16. Elliott J, Pedler A, Jull G, Van Wyk L, Galloway G, O'Leary S. Differential changes in muscle composition exist in traumatic and nontraumatic neck pain. Spine 2014;39(1):39–47.

17. Elliott J, Pedler A, Kenardy J, Galloway G, Jull G, Sterling M. The temporal development of fatty infiltrates in the neck muscles following whiplash injury: an association with pain and posttraumatic stress. PLoS One 2011;6(6):e21194.

18. Ferrari R, Russell A, Carroll L, Cassidy D. A re-examination of the whiplash associated disorders (WAD) as a systemic illness. Ann Rheum Dis 2005;64(9):1337–42.

19. Foa E. Posttraumatic stress diagnostic scale: manual. Minneapolis, MN: NCS Pearson; 1995.

20. Foa E, Cashman L, Jaycox L, Perry K. The validation of a self-report measure of posttraumatic stress disorder: the posttraumatic diagnostic scale. Psychol Assess 1997;9(4):445–51.

21. Gartner R, Jensen M, Nielsen J, Ewertz M, Kroman N, Kehlet H. Prevalance of an factors associated with persistent pain following breast cancer surgery. JAMA 2009;302(18):1985–92.

22. Goldsmith R, Wright C, Bell S, Rushton A. Cold hyperalgesia as a prognostic factor in whiplash associated disorders: a systematic review. Man Ther 2012;17(5):402–10.

23. Grant GM, O'Donnell ML, Spittal MJ, Creamer M, Studdert DM. Relationship between stressfulness of claiming for injury compensation and long-term recovery: a prospective cohort study. JAMA Psychiatry 2014;71(4):446–53.

24. Hanley M, Jensen M, Smith D, Ehde D, Edwards W, Robinson L. Preamputation pain and acute pain predcit chronic pain after lower extremity amputation. J Pain 2007;8(2):102–9.

25. Hill J, Whitehurst D, Lewis M, Bryan S, Dunn KM, Foster NE, Konstantinou K, Main CJ, Mason E, Somerville S, et al. Comparison of stratified primary care management for low back pain with current best practice (STarT Back): a randomised controlled trial. Lancet 2011;378:1560–71.

26. Holm L, Carroll L, Cassidy D, Skillgate E, Ahlbom A. Expectations for recovery important in the prognosis of whiplash injuries. PLoS Med 2008;5(5):e105.

27. Holme A, Williamson O, Hogg M, Arnold C, Prosser A, Clements J, Konstantatos A, O'Donnell M. Predictors of pain 12 months after serious injury. Pain Med 2010;11:1599–611.

28. Hunt M, Keefe F, Bryant C, Metcalf BR, Ahamed Y, Nicholas MK, Bennell KL. A physiotherapist-delivered, combined exercise and pain coping skills training intervention for individuals with knee osteoarthritis: a pilot study. Knee 2013;20:106–12.

29. Jenewein J, Wittmann L, Moergeli H, Creutzig J, Schnyder U. Mutual influence of PTSD symptoms and chronic pain among injred accident survivors: a longitudinal study. J Traumatic Stress 2009;22(6):540–8.

30. Johnston V, Jimmieson N, Jull G, Souvlis T. Quantitative sensory measures distinguish office workers with varying levels of neck pain and disability. Pain 2008;137:257–65.

31. Joslin C, Khan S, Bannister G. Long-term disability after neck injury. A comparative study. J Bone Joint Surg Br 2004;86(7):1032–4.

32. Jull G, Kenardy J, Hendrikz J, Cohen M, Sterling M. Management of acute whiplash: a randomized controlled trial of multidisciplinary stratified treatments. Pain 2013;154:1798–806.

33. Jull G, Trott P, Potter H, Zito G, Niere K, Shirley D, Emberson J, Marschner I, Richardson C. A randomised controlled trial of physiotherapy management for cervicogenic headache. Spine 2002;27(17):1835–43.

34. Kamper S, Rebbeck T, Maher C, McAuley J, Sterling M. Course and prognostic factors of whiplash: a systematic review and meta-analysis. Pain 2008;138(3):617–29.

35. Kasch H, Qerama E, Bach F, Jensen T. Reduced cold pressor pain tolerance in non-recovered whiplash patients: a 1 year prospective study. Eur J Pain 2005;9(5):561–9.

36. Kenardy J, Heron-Delaney M, Warren J, Brown EA. Effect of mental health on long-term disability after a road traffic crash: results from the UQ SuPPORT Study. Arch Phys Med Rehabil 2015; 96(3):410–7.

37. Kuch K, Cox B, Evans R, Shulman I. Phobias, panic and pain in 55 survivors of road vehicle accidents. J Anxiety Disord 1994;8(2):181–7.

38. Lamb S, Gates S, Williams MA, Williamson EM, Mt-Isa S, Withers EJ, Castelnuovo E, Smith J, Ashby D, Cooke MW, et al. Emergency department treatments and physiotherapy for acute whiplash: a pragmatic, two-step, randomised controlled trial. Lancet 2013;381(9866):546–56.

39. Lim E, Sterling M, Stone A, Vicenzino B. Central hyperexcitability as measured with nociceptive flexor reflex threshold in chronic musculoskeletal pain: a systematic review. Pain 2011;152(8):1811–20.

40. Mayou R, Bryant B. Psychiatry of whiplash neck injury. Br J Psychiatry 2002;180:441–8.

41. Michaleff Z, Maher C, Lin C, Rebbeck T, Connelly L, Jull G, Sterling M. Comprehensive physiotherapy exercise program or advice alone for chronic whiplash (PROMISE): a pragmatic randomised controlled trial (ACTRN12609000825257). Lancet 2014;384(9938):133–41.

42. Motor Accident Insurance Commission. Annual report 2011–2012. Brisbane: Motor Accident Insurance Commission; 2012.

43. Ng T, Pedler A, Vicenzino B, Sterling M. Less efficacious conditioned pain modulation and sensory hypersensitivity in chronic whiplash-associated disorders in Singapore. Clin J Pain 2014;30(5):436–42.

44. Ritchie C, Hendrikz J, Jull G, Elliott J, Sterling M. External validation of a clinical prediction rule to predict full recovery and continued moderate/severe disability following acute whiplash injury. J Orthop Sports Phys Ther 2015;45(4):242–50.

45. Ritchie C, Hendrikz J, Kenardy J, Sterling M. Development and validation of a screening tool to identify both chronicity and recovery following whiplash injury. Pain 2013;154:2198–206.

46. Scholten-Peeters GG, Verhagen AP, Bekkering GE, van der Windt DA, Barnsley L, Oostendorp RA, Hendriks EJ. Prognostic factors of whiplash associated disorders: a systematic review of prospective cohort studies. Pain 2003;104(1/2):303–22.

47. Scott D, Jull G, Sterling M. Widespread sensory hypersensitivity is a feature of chronic whiplash-associated disorder but not chronic idiopathic neck pain. Clin J Pain 2005;21(2):175–81.

48. Smith A, Jull G, Schneider G, Frizzell B, Hooper R, Sterling M. Cervical radiofrequency neurotomy reduces central hyperexcitability and improves neck movement in individuals with chronic whiplash. Pain Med 2014;15(1):128–41.

49. Spitzer WO, Skovron ML, Salmi LR, Cassidy JD, Duranceau J, Suissa S, Zeiss E. Scientific monograph of Quebec Task Force on whiplash associated disorders: redefining "whiplash" and its management. Spine 1995;20(8, Suppl):1S–73S.

50. Sterling M, Carroll L, Kasch H, Kamper S, Stemper B. Prognosis after whiplash injury: where to from here? Discussion Paper 3. Spine 2011;36(25, Suppl):S330–S334.

51. Sterling M, Elliott JM, Cabot PJ. The course of serum inflammatory biomarkers following whiplash injury and their relationship to sensory and muscle measures: a longitudinal cohort study. PLoS One 2013;8(10):e77903.

52. Sterling M, Hendrikz J, Kenardy J. Developmental trajectories of pain/disability and PTSD symptoms following whiplash injury. Pain 2010;150(1):22–8.

53. Sterling M, Hendrikz J, Kenardy J. Similar factors predict disability and PTSD trajectories following whiplash injury. Pain 2011;152(6):1272–8.

54. Sterling M, Hendrikz J, Kenardy J, Kristjansson E, Dumas JP, Niere K, Cote J, Deserres S, Rivest K, Jull G. Assessment and validation of prognostic models for poor functional recovery 12 months after whiplash injury: a multicentre inception cohort study. Pain 2012;153(8):1727–34.

55. Sterling M, Jull G, Kenardy J. Physical and psychological predictors of outcome following whiplash injury maintain predictive capacity at long term follow-up. Pain 2006;122:102–8.

56. Sterling M, Jull G, Vizenzino B, Kenardy J, Darnell R. Development of motor system dysfunction following whiplash injury. Pain 2003;103:65–73.

57. Sterling M, Jull G, Vicenzino B, Kenardy J, Darnell R. Physical and psychological factors predict outcome following whiplash injury. Pain 2005;114:141–8.

58. Stone A, Vicenzino B, Lim E, Sterling M. Measures of central hyperexcitability in chronic whiplash associated disorder—a systematic review and meta-analysis. Man Ther 2012;18(2):111–7.

59. Sullivan M, Adams H, Horan S, Maher D, Boland D, Gross R. The role of perceived injustice in the experience of chronic pain and disability: scale development and validation. J Occup Rehabil 2008;18:249–61.

60. Sullivan M, Stanish W, Waite H, Sullivan M, Tripp D. Catastrophizing, pain, and disability in patients with soft-tissue injuries. Pain 1998;77:253–60.

61. Sullivan M, Thibault P, Simmonds M, Milioto M, Cantin AP, Velly A. Pain, perceived injustice and the persistence of post-traumatic stress symptoms during the course of rehabilitation for whiplash injuries. Pain 2009;145(3):325–31.

62. Teasell RW, McClure JA, Walton D, Pretty J, Salter K, Meyer M, Sequeira K, Death B. A research synthesis of therapeutic interventions for whiplash-associated disorder (WAD), Part 2: interventions for acute WAD. Pain Res Manage 2010;15(5):295–304.

63. Teasell RW, McClure JA, Walton D, Pretty J, Salter K, Meyer M, Sequeira K, Death B. A research synthesis of therapeutic interventions for whiplash-associated disorder (WAD), Part 4: non invasive interventions for chronic WAD. Pain Res Manage 2010;15(5):313–22.

64. Treleaven J. Sensorimotor disturbances in neck disorders affecting postural stability, head and eye movement control. Man Ther 2008;13(1):2–11.

65. Turk D. The biopsychosocial approach to the assessment and intervention for people with musculoskeletal disorders. In: Gatchel R, Schultz I, editors. Handbook of musculoskeletal pain and disability disorders in the workplace. New York, NY: Springer; 2013. pp. 341–64.

66. Van Oosterwijck J, Nijs J, Meeus M, Paul L. Evidence for central sensitization in chronic whiplash: a systematic literature review. Eur J Pain 2013;17:299–312.

67. Vos T, Flaxman A, Naghavi M, Lozano R, Michaud C, Ezzati M, Shibuya K, Salomon JA, Abdalla S, Aboyans V, et al. Years lived with disability (YLDs) for 1160 sequelae of 289 diseases and injuries 1990–2010: a systematic analysis for the Global Burden of Disease Study 2010. Lancet 2012;380:2163–96.

68. Walton D, McDermid J, Teasell R, Nielson W, Reese H, Levesque L. Pressure pain threshold testing demonstrates predictive ability in people with acute whiplash. J Orthop Sports Phys Ther 2011;41(9):658–65.

69. Walton D, Pretty J, MacDermid J, Teasell R. Risk factors for persistent problems following whiplash injury: results of a systematic review and meta-analysis. J Orthop Sports Phys Ther 2009;39(5):334–50.

70. Williamson E, Williams M, Gates S, Lamb S. A systematic review of psychological factors and the development of late whiplash syndrome. Pain 2008;135:20–30.

CHAPTER 9

The Clinical Examination for Risk Factors in Whiplash Trauma

Helge Kasch

Attempts to classify whiplash (WL) patients in order to predict chronicity and long-term disability following trauma have been unsuccessful. Treatment studies applying the existing classification or grading systems even with individualized therapy have been unable to improve the outcome after WL injuries [30, 38].

Twenty years ago, The Quebec Task Force introduced the whiplash-associated disorders (WAD) grading system, with grades from 0 to IV based on encountered symptoms and neurological findings after exposure to a WL trauma. More recent WL literature rules out the WAD [34] grades 0 and IV as being WL injuries [3]. However, restricting the application of the WAD grading system to grades I–III has shown limited power as a tool for predicting the transition toward chronicity [25]. Recent research has emphasized the importance of both psychological and social factors in combination with the apparent biological features presented by the patient at first examination [1, 4, 5, 12, 31, 32].

Nociceptive sensitization is present in both acute and chronic WL patients. Nonrecovery is probably related to the initial pain barrage and to previous pain conditions, and may also be related to genetic factors [7, 8, 20]. Patients with initial moderate or severe headache or neck pain without previous pain had a fourfold higher risk of work disablement after 1 year, and patients with more than 14 days of minor headache/neck pain during the last year had a 2.5-fold higher risk [23]. An altered general response to cold pain 5 days after trauma may relate to genetic or pretrauma susceptibility of ascending and/or descending pathways for nociceptive sensitization, but for the time being this is only speculative.

Several clinical and epidemiological studies support pretrauma non-specific stress, depression, catastrophizing, expectation, future despair, and perceived injustice, and other psychological factors play a role for nonrecovery [3, 5, 14, 27, 32, 36, 37]. Psychological factors such as fear of movement, kinesophobia, catastrophizing, and coping strategies play a role in reduced neck mobility and nonrecovery, persistence, or worsening of pain [2, 31]. In similarity to the CROM test being a psychophysical test, many nonpainful symptoms may reflect both the severity of a physical injury and also the presence of bodily distress [10]. The role of the examiner, the therapist, as a fear-inducer has been debated [6, 37].

The initial evaluation of easily obtainable clinical parameters, including visual analogue scale (VAS) for neck pain and headache, and the number of nonpainful neurological symptoms and active neck mobility (cervical range of motion [CROM] [24]) is easily done at the first visit after WL trauma. From a clinical point of view, it is reasonable to stratify WL-exposed patients into different risk categories soon after exposure based on early clinical findings. We conducted two clinical prospective studies using clinical assessment and patient-reported symptoms with 12-year follow-up (Flowchart in Fig. 9-1) [18, 23].

First, we performed a 1-year observational study of 141 acute WL patients (WAD grade I–III) exposed to rear-end motor vehicle accident (MVA), and 40 sex-matched and age-matched controls exposed to acute nonsport ankle sprain. The two patient groups reported similar disability and global pain within the first week after trauma, but at 1 year posttrauma, only the WL patient group reported nonrecovery [18], whereas all ankle sprain patients recovered. Neurological examination was performed at the first visit. Semistructured interviews were conducted after 1 week, 1 month, and 3, 6, and 12 months following trauma. In addition, patients completed a set of self-reports, namely, The McGill Pain Questionnaire [9], the Danish version, The Millon Behavioral Health

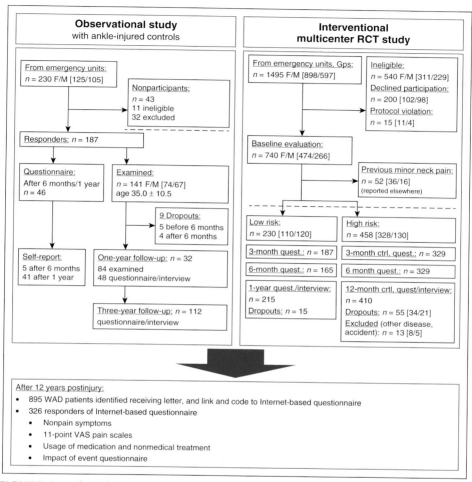

FIGURE 9-1 Flowchart of observational and interventional prospective whiplash studies.

Inventory [11], the symptom check list (SCL-90R), The Copenhagen Neck Functional Disability Scale [16]. We were particularly interested in the role of sensitization of the nociceptive system as a possible mechanism for development of long-term pain and disability. Therefore, we examined the development of the functioning of the diffuse noxious inhibitory control system in a cold pressor test [20] prospectively. We observed the development of remote and regional pain with pressure algometry detection and tolerance thresholds, and applied the methodical palpation technique in the neck and jaw muscles of the WL patients and controls [29]. We measured active neck mobility (CROM test [24]), and maximal voluntary contraction and duration for neck flexion and neck extension. In a second study, we performed a multicenter interventional randomized trial of 740 acute WL patients divided into high- and low-risk strata based on risk factors derived from the former observational study [18, 23]. The derived risk factors from the former study were: (1) intense initial neck pain or headache, (2) multiple nonpainful neurological symptoms, and (3) reduced active neck mobility from early aftertrauma (median 4.5 days after trauma). These factors were used for an algorithm to classify patients in the treatment study into either a low-risk or a high-risk group. (For details on the intervention study results refer to [23, 28].) High-risk patients had a 10-fold raised risk of 1-year work disability. However, these factors do not reveal the mechanisms responsible for chronic disability after WL trauma, but merely allude to the multifaceted nature of disability in WAD.

RISK STRATA

The risk score we identified and described above was robust in predicting 1-year work disability (Fig. 9-2), revealing receiver operating characteristic (ROC) curve areas of 0.89 in the first study. Furthermore, in the second multicenter study, we had several examiners assessing acute whiplash patients with above risk-factors. ROC curve areas of 0.87 showed robustness of the risk score [19, 22].

From a clinical perspective, we found it meaningful when examining data in both studies to segregate the risk score into seven risk strata, and Table 9-1 provides detailed information on risk score and grading.

Fig. 9-3 shows that WL-associated symptoms are very differently distributed in the seven risk strata 12 years after exposure to WL trauma.

DESCRIPTORS OF PAIN AND CLINICAL CORRELATES OF PAIN

The risk strata we identified were nicely supported by the McGill Pain Questionnaire (see Fig. 9-4E), with P values below 0.004 (Kruskal Wallis); the number of pain descriptive words count (NWC) was

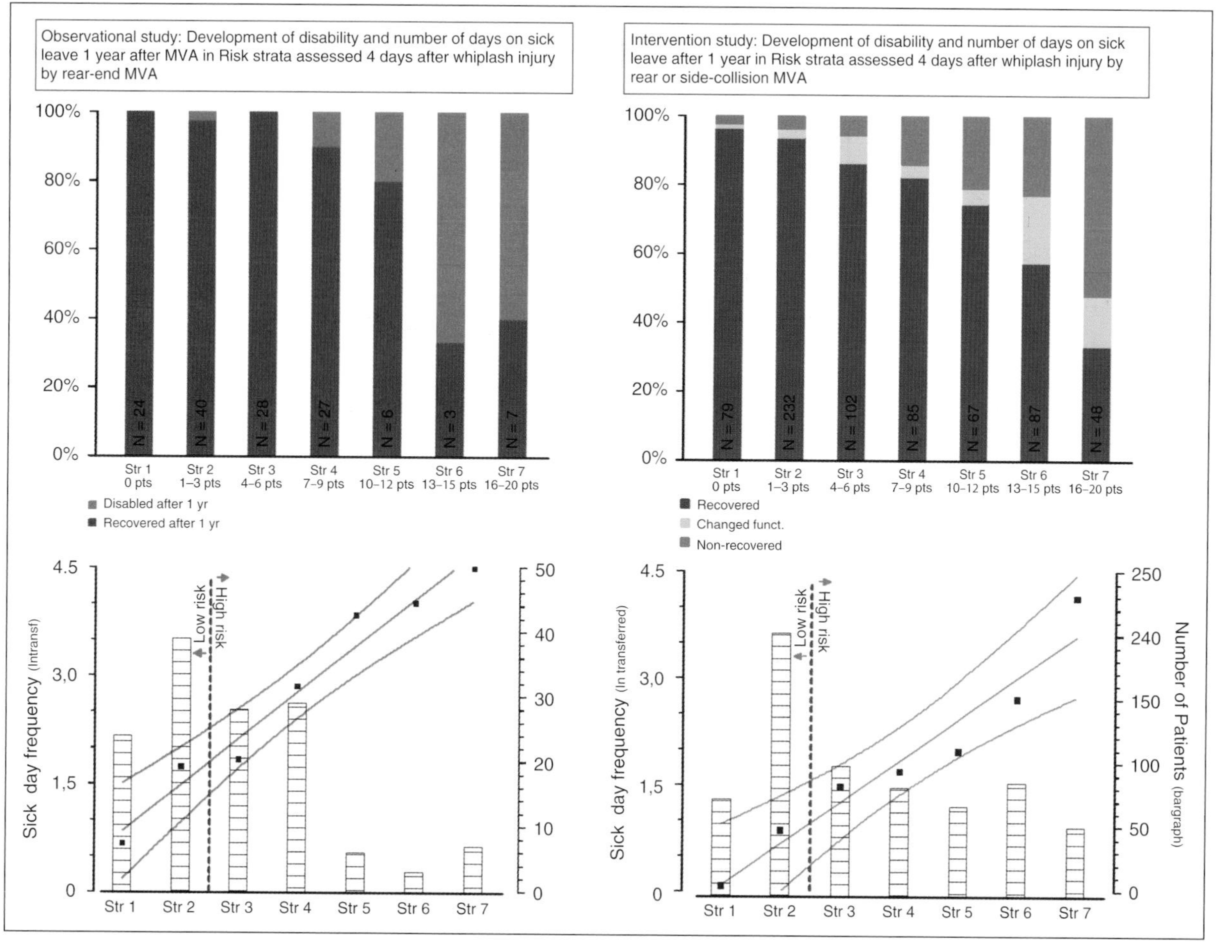

FIGURE 9-2 Column 1 shows development of work disability after 1 year and number of days on sick leave (ln transformed) during first year after injury in observational study in seven risk strata. Column 2 shows development of work disability, changed functioning after 1 year in interventional study, and number of days on sick leave (ln transformed) during first year in seven risk strata.

145

TABLE 9-1 The Danish Whiplash Study Group Risk Assessment Score

Points	0	1	2	3	4	5	6	7	8	9	10
CROM	>280		261–280		241–260		221–240		200–220		<200
Neck/Head VAS	0–2	3–4			5–8		9–10				
Number of nonpain symptoms		3–5		6–11							

Note: Stratum 1 = 0 pts; Stratum 2 = 1–3 pts; Stratum 3 = 4–6 pts; Stratum 4 = 7–9 pts; Stratum 5 = 10–12 pts; Stratum 6 = 13–15 pts; Stratum 7 = 16–19 pts.

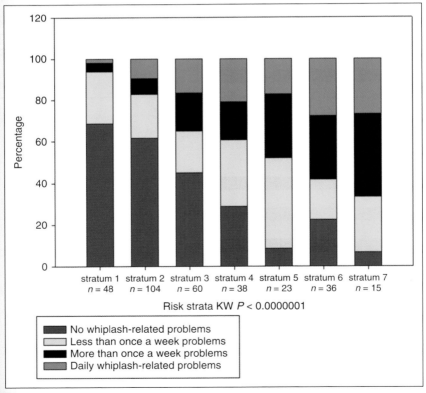

FIGURE 9-3 Frequency of whiplash-related symptoms reported after 12 years in seven risk strata with stratification made 4 days after WL trauma exposure.

significantly raised in higher risk strata ($P < 0.0001$). The trajectory for each stratum in Fig. 9-4A–D shows good long-term differentiation between lines for both neck pain (Fig. 9-4A), headache (Fig. 9-4B), and work-related issues (Fig. 9-4C and D). Tenderness of muscles assessed by pressure algometry (Somedic Algometer 1, $P < 0.002$), methodical palpation [29] ($P < 1.78 \times 10^{-6}$), and time to peak pain during the cold pressor test ($P < 0.01$) were also distributed in concordance with the Risk Assessment Score [22]. Voluntary neck muscle strength examination (see Fig. 9-4G) of maximal voluntary contraction (MVC), using the Follo Neck Exercizer, Norway, was concordant

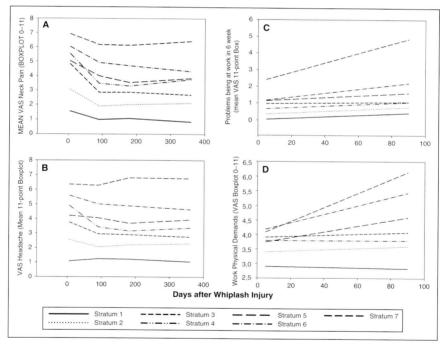

FIGURE 9-4 A: Development of neck pain intensity (VAS 0–10) in interventional study during 1-year observation in seven risk strata. **B:** Development of headache intensity (VAS 0–10) in interventional study during 1-year observation in seven risk strata. **C:** Development of expectancy of work-related problems in next 6 weeks (VAS 0–10) in interventional study during 100 days of observation in seven risk strata. **D:** Development of evaluation of the physical demands of job (VAS 0–10) in interventional study during 100 days of observation in seven risk strata. (*continued*)

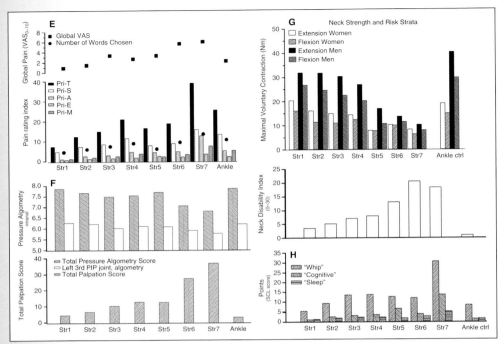

FIGURE 9-4 (*continued*) **E:** Initial mean global pain (VAS 0–10) and Pain Rating Index (McGill Pain Questionnaire) in seven risk strata of acute whiplash trauma patients and acute ankle-injured controls in the observational study during first week. **F:** Deep muscle pain assessed with pressure algometry (total neck and jaw muscle score), (pressure pain detection thresholds), and (peripheral score of joint left 3rd finger PIP joint) and methodic palpation total score of neck and jaw muscles in seven risk strata of acute whiplash trauma patients and acute ankle-injured controls in the observational study during first week. **G:** Strength obtained in triplicates of neck extension and neck flexion a.m. Jordan et al. [17] in seven risk strata of acute whiplash trauma patients, and acute ankle-injured controls divided by gender in the observational study during first week. **H:** Score on 15-item (0–45) The Copenhagen Neck Functional Disability Scale [16] in whiplash patients in seven risk strata and ankle-injured controls after 1 week and below score on WHIP, COGN, and morning SLEEP parameters in seven risk strata and ankle-injured controls.

with risk strata for both neck flexion (split by gender, $P < 0.001$) and neck extension ($P < 0.004$), and duration of 60% of MVC for flexion ($P < 0.001$) and extension ($P < 0.001$) as well [17]. The Copenhagen Neck Disability Index score [16] obtained 1 week after trauma fitted well with the risk strata ($P < 0.002$) (Fig. 9-4H). From the symptom

checklist SCL-90R, the WHIP, COGN, and morning SLEEP[1] parameters were obtained, as described by Smed [33], and higher WHIP
scores, but also scores on cognitive and sleep problems, were found in
higher risk strata after 3 months.

DISCUSSION

Data from these clinical measurements are as biological means in concordance with the aforementioned stratification. Psychophysical tests
such as the cold pressor test, pressure algometry in remote area and in
neck vicinity, and tenderness assessed by means of the Langemark and
Olesen method for methodical palpation [29] showed significant difference in strata. Flexion and extension neck muscle strength and duration
were also a psychophysical measure that was well distributed according
to risk strata. The predictive value of the CROM test has been supported
only in some prospective studies [3, 38]. In both studies conducted
by The Danish Whiplash Study Group, patients with reduced CROM
($<240°$) had a 4.5-fold greater risk of work disablement after 1 year. In
these studies, CROM was the most important factor in the risk score.
The background for reduced neck mobility may reflect a kyphotic neck
stature, which was associated with neck pain; however, this did not relate to recovery in 171 acute MRI-scanned WL patients [15]. Using nee-
dle electromyography, the author has identified more than 200 chronic
and 30 subacute (<1 week after trauma) WL patients having dystonic
features in neck muscles (i.e., splenius capitis, semispinalis, scalenus and
splenius cervicis, and longisssimus dorsi muscles). Dystonic features in
the neck may contribute to reduced neck mobility (but also pain, distress, proprioceptive malfunctioning, dizziness, and sleep disturbance).
The role of dystonic EMG pattern after WL is not clear yet.

---

[1] WHIP consists of 5 symptoms: 4/12 symptoms of the SOM scale—headache, back pain,
muscle pain, numbness, and paresthesia—and 1/10 of the PSYscale: "fear of something
serious being wrong with the body." COGN consists of 5 symptoms all from the Obsessive-
Compulsive scale: concentration and memory trouble, mind going blank, having to check
and slow down. SLEEP consists of trouble falling asleep, awakening early in the morning,
restless or disturbed.

CONCLUSIONS

In clinical studies of WL injuries, the initial pain intensity, the degree of nociceptive sensitization, and the presence of a set of psychological risk factors have shown predictive value for nonrecovery after acute WL trauma by other research groups [13, 26, 35] and from our studies summarized above [5, 20, 21, 27]. Clinical assessment with grading WL patients by means of (a) active neck mobility in 6 defined directions, (b) VAS pain score of combined headache and neck pain in conjunction with (c) sum of selected nonpainful symptoms is easily obtained in a unit, or by the general practitioner or physiotherapist or manual therapist, and combined into a risk score and following risk stratum. We propose that The Danish Whiplash Study Group Risk Assessment Score, now showing 12 years' durability of predicting disability and pain after acute WL trauma (Fig. 9-3), as explained in this chapter, should be applied for future stratification of WL patients in the clinic and for future WL research. This model seems to fulfill a need for bio-psychosocial robustness in order to predict patient trajectories after WL. There is a need for identifying patients at risk for nonrecovery at an early point, and this could be of essence in the need for future treatment studies for both acute and chronic WL patients.

REFERENCES

1. Boersma K, Linton SJ. Expectancy, fear and pain in the prediction of chronic pain and disability: a prospective analysis. Eur J Pain 2006;10(6):551–7.

2. Buitenhuis J, Jaspers JP, Fidler V. Can kinesiophobia predict the duration of neck symptoms in acute whiplash? Clin J Pain 2006;22(3):272–7.

3. Carroll LJ, Hogg-Johnson S, Côté P, van der Velde G, Holm LW, Carragee EJ, Hurwitz EL, Peloso PM, Cassidy JD, Guzman J, et al. Course and prognostic factors for neck pain in workers: results of the Bone and Joint Decade 2000–2010 Task Force on Neck Pain and Its Associated Disorders. J Manipulative Physiol Ther 2009;32(2, Suppl):S108–S116.

4. Carstensen TB. The influence of psychosocial factors on recovery following acute whiplash trauma. Dan Med J 2012;59(12):B4560.

5. Carstensen TB, Frostholm L, Oernboel E, Kongsted A, Kasch H, Jensen TS, Fink P. Post-trauma ratings of pre-collision pain and psychological distress predict

poor outcome following acute whiplash trauma: a 12-month follow-up study. Pain 2008;139(2):248–59.

6. Cote P, Hogg-Johnson S, Cassidy JD, Carroll L, Frank JW, Bombardier C. Early aggressive care and delayed recovery from whiplash: isolated finding or reproducible result? Arthritis Rheum 2007;57(5):861–8.

7. Curatolo M, Petersen-Felix S, Arendt-Nielsen L, Giani C, Zbinden A, Radanov B. Central hypersensitivity in chronic pain after whiplash injury. Clin J Pain 2001;17(4): 306–15.

8. Diatchenko L, Nackley AG, Slade GD, Fillingim RB, Maixner W. Idiopathic pain disorders—pathways of vulnerability. Pain 2006;123(3):226–30.

9. Drewes AM, Helweg-Larsen S, Petersen P, Brennum J, Andreasen A, Poulsen LH. McGill Pain Questionaire translated into Danish: experimental and clinical findings. Clin J Pain 1993;9(2):80–7.

10. Fink P, Rosendal M. Recent developments in the understanding and management of functional somatic symptoms in primary care. Curr Opin Psychiatry 2008;21(2): 182–8.

11. Gatchel RJ, Deckel AW, Weinberg N, Smith JE. The utility of the Millon Behavioral Health Inventory in the study of chronic headaches. Headache 1985;25(49):49–54.

12. Gehrt TB, Wisbech Carstensen TB, Ornbol E, Fink PK, Kasch H, Frostholm L. The role of illness perceptions in predicting outcome after acute whiplash trauma: a multicenter 12-month follow-up study. Clin J Pain 2015;31(1):14–20.

13. Graven-Nielsen T, Curatolo M, Mense S. Central sensitization, referred pain, and deep tissue hyperalgesia in musculoskeletal pain. In: Flor H, Kalso E, Dostrovsky JO, editors. Proceedings of the 11th World Congress on Pain. Seattle, WA: IASP Press; 2006. pp. 217–30.

14. Holm LW, Carroll LJ, Cassidy JD, Skillgate E, Ahlbom A. Expectations for recovery important in the prognosis of whiplash injuries. PLoS Med 2008;5(5):e105.

15. Johansson MP, Baann Liane MS, Bendix T, Kasch H, Kongsted A. Does cervical kyphosis relate to symptoms following whiplash injury? Man Ther 2011;16(4):378–83.

16. Jordan A, Manniche C, Mosdal C, Hindsberger C. The Copenhagen Neck Functional Disability Scale: a study of reliability and validity. J Manipulative Physiol Ther 1998;21(8):520–7.

17. Jordan A, Mehlsen J, Bulow PM, Ostergaard K, Danneskiold-Samsoe B. Maximal isometric strength of the cervical musculature in 100 healthy volunteers. Spine (Phila Pa 1976) 1999;24(13):1343–8.

18. Kasch H, Bach FW, Jensen TS. Handicap after acute whiplash injury: a 1-year prospective study of risk factors. Neurology 2001;56(12):1637–43.

19. Kasch H, Kongsted A, Qerama E, Bach FW, Bendix T, Jensen TS. A new stratified risk assessment tool for whiplash injuries developed from a prospective observational study. BMJ Open 2013;3(1):e002050.

20. Kasch H, Qerama E, Bach FW, Jensen TS. Reduced cold pressor pain tolerance in non-recovered whiplash patients: a 1-year prospective study. Eur J Pain 2005;9(5):561–9.

21. Kasch H, Qerama E, Kongsted A, Bach FW, Bendix T, Jensen TS. Deep muscle pain, tender points and recovery in acute whiplash patients: a 1-year follow-up study. Pain 2008;140(1):65–73.

22. Kasch H, Qerama E, Kongsted A, Bach FW, Bendix T, Jensen TS. The risk assessment score in acute whiplash injury predicts outcome and reflects bio-psycho-social factors. Spine (Phila Pa 1976) 2011;36(25, Suppl):S263–S267.

23. Kasch H, Qerama E, Kongsted A, Bendix T, Jensen TS, Bach FW. Clinical assessment of prognostic factors for long-term pain and handicap after whiplash injury: a 1-year prospective study. Eur J Neurol 2008;15(11):1222–30.

24. Kasch H, Stengaard-Pedersen K, Arendt-Nielsen L, Staehelin Jensen T. Headache, neck pain, and neck mobility after acute whiplash injury: a prospective study. Spine (Phila Pa 1976) 2001;26(11):1246–51.

25. Kivioja J, Lindgren U, Jensen I. A prospective study on the Quebec Classification as a predictor for the outcome after whiplash injury. World Congress Whiplash Associated Disorders. Vancouver, Canada; February 1999. p. 131.

26. Koelbaek Johansen M, Graven-Nielsen T, Schou-Olesen A, Arendt-Nielsen L. Generalised muscular hyperalgesia in chronic whiplash syndrome. Pain 1999;83(1):229–34.

27. Kongsted A, Bendix T, Qerama E, Kasch H, Bach FW, Korsholm L, Jensen TS. Acute stress response and recovery after whiplash injuries. A one-year prospective study. Eur J Pain 2008;12(4):455–63.

28. Kongsted A, Qerama E, Kasch H, Bendix T, Bach FW, Korsholm L, Jensen TS. Neck collar, "act-as-usual" or active mobilization for whiplash injury? A randomized parallel-group trial. Spine (Phila Pa 1976) 2007;32(6):618–26.

29. Langemark M, Olesen J. Pericranial tenderness in tension headache. Cephalalgia 1987;7:249–55.

30. Michaleff ZA, Maher CG, Lin CW, Rebbeck T, Jull G, Latimer J, Connelly L, Sterling M. Comprehensive physiotherapy exercise programme or advice for chronic whiplash (PROMISE): a pragmatic randomised controlled trial. Lancet 2014;384(9938):133–41.

31. Myrtveit SM, Carstensen T, Kasch H, Ornbol E, Frostholm L. Initial healthcare and coping preferences are associated with outcome 1 year after whiplash trauma: a multi-centre 1-year follow-up study. BMJ Open 2015;5(3):e007239.

32. Robinson JP, Burwinkle T, Turk DC. Perceived and actual memory, concentration, and attention problems after whiplash-associated disorders (grades I and II): prevalence and predictors. Arch Phys Med Rehabil 2007;88(6):774–9.

33. Smed A. Cognitive function and distress after common whiplash injury. Acta Neurol Scand 1997;95:73–80.

34. Spitzer WO, Skovron ML, Salmi LR, Cassidy JD, Duranceau J, Suissa S, Zeiss E. Scientific monograph of the Quebec Task Force on whiplash-associated disorders: redefining "whiplash" and it's management. Spine 1995;20(8, Suppl):1S–73S.

35. Sterling M, Jull G, Vicenzino B, Kenardy J, Darnell R. Physical and psychological factors predict outcome following whiplash injury. Pain 2005;114:141–8.

36. Vangronsveld K, Peters M, Goossens M, Linton S, Vlaeyen J. Applying the fear-avoidance model to the chronic whiplash syndrome. Pain 2007;131(3):258–61.

37. Vlaeyen JW, Linton SJ. Are we "fear-avoidant"? Pain 2006;124(3):240–1.

38. Walton DM, Carroll LJ, Kasch H, Sterling M, Verhagen AP, Macdermid JC, Gross A, Santaguida PL, Carlesso L; International Collaboration on Neck Pain. An Overview of Systematic Reviews on Prognostic Factors in Neck Pain: results from the International Collaboration on Neck Pain (ICON) Project. Open Orthop J 2013;7:494–505.

CHAPTER 10

Neurobiological Mechanisms of Whiplash

Samuel A. McLean

Among individuals involved in one of the fifty million motor vehicle collisions (MVCs) that occur worldwide each year [37], persistent musculoskeletal pain is a common and costly public health problem [7]. The purpose of this chapter is to provide a contemporary understanding of neurobiological mechanisms mediating persistent symptom development after MVC. The past two decades have witnessed the increasing application of molecular techniques to gain insight into the pathogenesis of post-MVC pain. However, the most important advance in understanding neurobiological mechanisms mediating post-MVC pain outcomes has been the evolution to a more accurate and complete characterization of the phenotype. This is of critical importance because if the phenotype is not accurately characterized, then it is unlikely that any amount of application of bioinformatic, statistical, or "omics" techniques will yield valid information. Candidate neurobiological systems responsible for the pathogenesis of post-MVC neuropsychiatric sequelae will then be reviewed, with an emphasis on those domains most fruitful for future study.

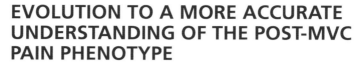

EVOLUTION TO A MORE ACCURATE UNDERSTANDING OF THE POST-MVC PAIN PHENOTYPE

From Neck Pain to Neck Region Pain with Associated Symptoms

Studies of pain after MVC dating from as early as the 1950s focused on pain in the neck region [19], and cases of post-MVC pain were attributed to "whiplash injury" of the neck [19, 23, 40]. Consistent with this hypothesis, studies evaluating neurobiological mechanisms of post-MVC pain pathogenesis focused almost exclusively on the neck. In 1995, the Quebec Task Force on Whiplash-Associated Disorders changed the term from whiplash to "Whiplash-Associated Disorders" [42]. This change in terminology was made because (1) it was recognized that pain was not limited to the neck region (although additional areas of pain were believed to be limited to adjacent regions), and (2) it had become apparent that not only pain but also cognitive and somatic symptoms were frequent components of the syndrome [42]. (Of note, the association between cognitive symptoms and head injury has been shown to be extremely weak [8].) Even after the Quebec Task Force, most of the research into biological mechanisms mediating persistent post-MVC pain continued to be based on the hypothesis that biological mechanisms mediating post-MVC pain were due to neck injury during MVC.

From Pain in the Neck Region to Pain Potentially Occurring in Many Body Regions as Part of a Frequently Multidimensional Posttraumatic Neuropsychiatric Disorder

More recently, large-scale studies have shown that pain after MVC may occur in many different body regions (e.g., low back [9]), and/or may be widespread [25, 26, 50, 51]. For example, in one recent study of 948 individuals enrolled in the emergency department (ED) in the immediate aftermath of MVC, pain outside of the neck region at the time of ED evaluation was the norm, and 22% had pain in 7 or more body regions

[33]. At 6 weeks, moderate or severe low back pain was as common as neck pain (with a prevalence of 37% for each) and overlapped with neck pain in only 23% of patients [4]. Further, pain across all body regions accounted for nearly twice as much of the variance in pain interference as neck pain alone (60% vs. 34%). Similarly, in two large cohorts of individuals experiencing MVC who presented to the ED after MVC and were discharged to home after evaluation, 6 weeks after MVC, 528/859 (61.5%) of European Americans reported MVC-related pain outside body areas considered "whiplash-related" (head, neck, shoulders, and upper back), and 562/668 (84.1%) of African Americans reported pain outside such areas (unpublished data). Together, these data demonstrate that pain in body regions other than "whiplash-associated disorders" regions are very common after MVC and contribute substantially to overall pain-related disability. Thus, evaluating neck pain alone poorly characterizes the patient's pain experience. Along with these increasing data that pain often occurs across many regions after MVC, and is frequently widespread, evidence has also continued to accrue that post-MVC pain often occurs in the context of other symptoms. For example, Dr. Michele Sterling and others have shown that pain after MVC, and PTSD symptoms after MVC are often comorbid [17, 44, 45], and depressive symptoms have also been shown to be frequently comorbid with post-MVC pain [6, 22, 35], along with a wide variety of somatic symptoms [36].

While patients experience coincident pain and somatic and/or psychological symptoms as part of one syndrome, most patients have each symptom type evaluated independently in compartmentalized, siloed clinical settings. An individual with persistent symptoms after MVC might, for example, see a psychiatrist for an evaluation of posttraumatic stress disorder and/or depressive symptoms, a neurologist for somatic symptoms labeled as "postconcussive," and a physiatrist or anesthesiology pain medicine specialist for posttraumatic musculoskeletal pain. Similarly, research into biological mechanisms has also often been compartmentalized, with outcomes focused on one symptom domain or another. Better aligning neurobiological studies with the patient experience, by evaluating individuals according to multidimensional symptom cluster trajectory rather than symptom component, would allow us to most accurately assess the neurobiological substrate of different multidimensional post-MVC syndromes.

CANDIDATE BIOLOGICAL MECHANISMS MEDIATING POST-MVC OUTCOMES

Tissue Injury to Neck Structures

As described above, consistent with the pathophysiologic hypothesis that persistent symptoms after MVC result from abnormal neck motion, most studies evaluating neurobiological mechanisms of post-MVC pain pathogenesis have focused on the neck. A peripheral nociceptive input is capable of dynamically maintaining chronic pain over a broader local area [21]; tissue structures that might provide an ongoing source of nociceptive input are many, including the zygapophysial joint capsule, anuli fibrosi, and various ligaments, muscles, and intra-articular structures [12]. The best studied of these candidate structures is the zygapophysial joint. A small randomized controlled trial of radiofrequency neurotomy of zygapophysial joint cervical medial branch nerves in 24 patients with chronic neck pain after MVC found that the intervention group had substantially improved neck pain outcomes. In addition, several small, nonrandomized observational case series also suggest a potential treatment benefit [1, 30]. A transient peripheral tissue injury might also result in the development of persistent post-MVC pain, if this transient injury caused peripheral and/or central sensitization that then became self-sustaining. Whether such a phenomenon accounts for persistent post-MVC pain development in some individuals is unknown.

These data suggest that peripheral tissue injury may contribute to chronic post-MVC pain in some individuals. However, as already described, important features of common post-MVC symptom phenotypes are poorly explained by cervicogenic mechanisms, including the typical occurrence of pain in body regions distant from the neck, the common prevalence of widespread pain, and the often multidimensional nature of the phenotype, of which pain symptoms are only one part. In addition, if injury-related damage to cervical structures occurring at the moment of MVC played a dominant role in the genesis of post-MVC pain symptoms, then in epidemiologic studies, collision-related characteristics (e.g., vehicle speed, direction of collision, amount of vehicle damage) would be expected to be important risk factors for chronic post-MVC pain development. In study after study, however, collision-related factors have consistently been shown to be poor predictors of post-MVC pain outcomes [3, 6, 7, 10, 11, 17, 24, 26, 33, 44, 45]. Biomechanical experts frequently argue that this lack of association is due to the inability of epidemiologic studies to capture all of the subtleties of individual crash histories, such as the degree of neck flexion or extension at the moment of impact, the degree of lateral rotation of the neck at the moment of impact, and the distance of the head from the car head restraint. This is not a valid reason to discount epidemiologic study results, however, for while no study evaluates every potentially relevant variable, unless a consistent relationship exists between an important unmeasured third variable and measured variable(s), the relationship between the measured variable and outcome is unaffected. For example, cigarette smoking has consistently been shown to be a dominant risk factor for lung cancer development even though epidemiologic studies identifying this association have never accounted for all of the subtleties of individual cigarette smoking histories, such as cigarette brand, proportion of time spent smoking indoors versus outdoors, method of holding cigarette and inhaling, proportion of time that smoker tends to leave cigarette burning in ashtray versus smoking, secondhand smoke exposure, etc. If MVC-related tissue injury played a central role in the pathogenesis of post-MVC pain, then collision-related factors should be dominant predictors of pain outcomes. But they are not.

Other lines of evidence also suggest that MVC-related tissue injury does not play a central role in the neurobiological changes causing persistent post-MVC pain. There is great variation in the prevalence of chronic pain following MVC between different populations [18], and collisions that occur in other environmental settings (e.g., carnival "bumper cars") appear to exert the same biomechanical stress as a low-speed MVC, yet prolonged pain after bumper car collision is rare [10]. The study of Castro et al. [11], in which participants were exposed to a "sham" (placebo) rear-end collision, provides an extreme example of the disconnect between MVC characteristics and post-MVC pain symptoms. Twenty percent of participants reported pain and other symptoms 3 days after "sham" rear-end collision even though no actual collision occurred [11].

Another example of the disconnect between injury mechanism and persistent pain outcomes can be found by comparing the distribution of musculoskeletal pain symptoms among two groups of individuals who experienced two very different types of trauma: MVC and sexual assault [33, 46]. The MVC group consisted of 948 individuals who sought treatment from the ED after MVC and were discharged to home after evaluation. More than half of these individuals had severe damage to their vehicle, and more than half were transported to the ED by ambulance [33]. The sexual assault group consisted of 83 individuals who sought emergency care after being sexually assaulted. These women most often reported no extragenital physical trauma. Despite marked differences in type of tissue trauma experienced by these two groups, the distribution of pain experienced in many body regions, including axial regions, in the two groups 6 weeks after exposure was similar (Fig. 10-1).

Together, the above data provide only limited support for the hypothesis that neurobiological mechanisms resulting from tissue injury to neck structures are the primary cause of post-MVC pain symptoms. These data also suggest that the continued investigation of neurobiological mechanisms related to tissue injury is unlikely to be of great value to patients. The continued accumulation of data refuting a dominant role for tissue injury factors has created a void in understanding that, unfortunately, has often been filled with assumptions by caregivers, policymakers, and insurers that any individual with persistent post-MVC symptoms is malingering for financial gain, desire for opioid medication, etc. However, such assumptions ignore the potential role of stress and neuroimmune systems in contributing to the pathogenesis of persistent post-MVC pain.

Stress and Neuroimmune System Interactions

The pioneering pain researcher Dr. Patrick Wall conceptualized postinjury pain as part of a well-choreographed, time-dependent, integrated physiologic response whose purpose is to maximize the likelihood of

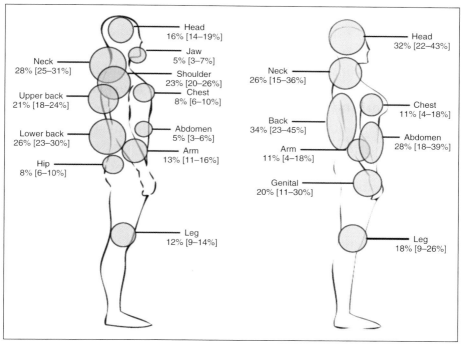

FIGURE 10-1 Areas of moderate or severe pain 6 weeks after motor vehicle collision (MVC), and areas of clinically significant new or worsening pain 6 weeks after sexual assault. Despite marked differences in injury mechanism and how pain regions were categorized, pain distributions in many regions, including axial regions, are similar. (Reproduced from McLean et al. [33] and from Ulirsch et al. [46].)

surviving a life threat [49]. Consistent with this hypothesis, subsequent decades of research have elucidated mechanisms by which the activation of stress systems such as endogenous opioid systems, catecholaminergic systems, and the hypothalamic–pituitary–adrenocortical axis exert time-dependent effects on memory [15], psychological responses [31, 38], wound healing [48], and metabolism [29] in a time-dependent and sometimes sex-dependent [2, 14] manner. Importantly, none of these effects depend on the presence of a tissue lesion. Rather, they are caused by neurobiological changes induced by the stress exposure itself. Similarly, increasing evidence suggests that these same physiologic systems contribute to the development of acute and persistent pain after MVC. Epidemiologic data supporting the involvement of such systems in the pathogenesis of post-MVC pain include data that vulnerability to post-MVC pain and psychological sequelae is shared and evidence that psychological symptoms known to be mediated by stress and neuroimmune system interactions predict post-MVC pain outcomes (for review see [15, 49]).

The results of recent candidate gene association studies also support the involvement of stress and neuroimmune system interactions in the pathogenesis of post-MVC pain. The utility of genetic association studies is that if a genetic variant is known to affect the function of a specific biological system or pathway, and that system is involved in the development of post-MVC pain, then the presence or absence of the genetic variant should be associated with vulnerability to develop post-MVC pain. Thus, association studies can test the hypothesis that a specific physiologic system is involved in the pathogenesis of post-MVC pain. Of note, genetic association studies for complex phenotypes such as post-MVC pain do not provide information regarding the degree of contribution of the physiologic system to post-MVC pain. This is because there are a great many genetic polymorphisms that, in aggregate, affect the function of the system, while in genetic association studies, only one or a small subset of genes is assessed.

Recent candidate gene studies have implicated the hypothalamic–pituitary–adrenal axis, catecholaminergic systems, opioid systems, and dopaminergic systems in the pathogenesis of post-MVC pain outcomes [2, 5, 28, 32, 39, 47]. Further evidence supporting the role of stress systems in the pathogenesis of persistent post-MVC pain comes from a recent study that evaluated the influence of living in a lower socioeconomic status neighborhood on post-MVC pain [47]. Living in a lower socioeconomic status neighborhood is known to cause alterations in stress system function [34, 41] (e.g., dysregulated cortisol levels [16, 27]). Even after adjusting for an array of individual-level factors, living in a lower socioeconomic status neighborhood was associated with worse pain outcomes [47]. Importantly, the adverse effect of living in a lower socioeconomic status neighborhood was evident only among those with genetic vulnerability to stress-induced pain (Fig. 10-2) [47].

Evidence for the importance of interactions between stress and neuroimmune systems in the pathogenesis of post-MVC pain also comes from a study by Sterling and colleagues [43]. These authors found circulating inflammatory markers in the early aftermath of MVC among

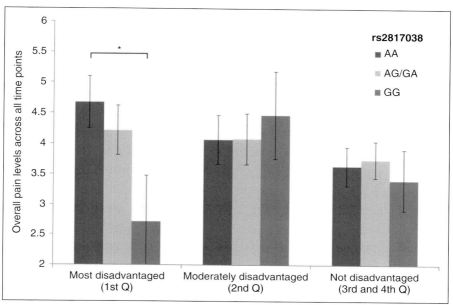

FIGURE 10-2 Gene-by-environment interaction between genetic vulnerability to stress-induced pain (single nucleotide polymorphism rs2817038 in the gene coding for cochaperone FK506 binding protein 51 [*FKBP5*]) and the most disadvantaged quartile (1st quartile) of neighborhood socioeconomic status. Error bars represent 95% confidence intervals of the least squares means. *Differences in overall pain among the genotypes is significant ($P < 0.0001$). MAF, minor allele frequency. (Reproduced from Ulirsch et al. *Pain* 2014.)

individuals with acute post-MVC pain, which persisted at 3 months only among those with continued pain [43]. The results of the above studies are consistent with a great deal of additional data from both preclinical and clinical studies that stress and neuroimmune systems play a critical role in the initiation and maintenance of many chronic pain states (for reviews contemporary at the time of press see [13, 20]).

CONCLUSIONS AND FUTURE DIRECTIONS

During the past two decades, the most important advance in understanding neurobiological mechanisms mediating post-MVC pain outcomes has, paradoxically, been not the application of the latest "omic" techniques, but rather a better characterization of the post-MVC pain phenotype. Individuals developing persistent pain after MVC have been shown to commonly experience pain across many body areas outside "whiplash areas," which is poorly predicted by collision characteristics. In addition, such pain symptoms are frequently only one component of a multidimensional syndrome characterized not only by pain symptoms but also by a range of other somatic and psychological symptoms. To help ensure that the full post-MVC symptom phenotype is evaluated in future studies, the field would benefit from replacing the term "whiplash-associated disorders" with a more general term such as "post-MVC neuropsychiatric sequelae." This might help to remove lingering misunderstanding among researchers and clinicians that pain symptoms occur in the neck region alone, and would avoid terms in the syndrome description that suggest a pathophysiologic mechanism with little supporting evidence. In addition, such a term would hopefully help advance the identification of common clusters of post-MVC symptoms (e.g., high pain, high somatic, low posttraumatic stress symptom cluster, high pain, low somatic, high posttraumatic stress symptom cluster, etc.).

Improved understanding of the post-MVC symptom phenotype, coincident with burgeoning evidence implicating stress and neuroimmune systems in both post-MVC pain and in a range of neuropsychiatric illnesses has resulted in these systems becoming leading candidate systems mediating the development of post-MVC neuropsychiatric sequelae. The role of such systems is supported by the results of candidate gene studies and ongoing molecular biological studies. Much more work to evaluate the role of these and other candidate neurobiological mechanisms is needed, so that the pathophysiology of specific clusters of multidimensional post-MVC neuropsychiatric syndromes can be defined. This work is critically important, because only by elucidating pathogenesis can optimal secondary preventive interventions be identified.

FUNDING

Research reported in this publication was supported by Award Numbers R01-AR056328, R01-AR064700, and R01-AR060852 from the National Institutes of Health. The content is solely the responsibility of the author and does not necessarily represent the official views of the National Institutes of Health.

REFERENCES

1. Barnsley L. Percutaneous radiofrequency neurotomy for chronic neck pain: outcomes in a series of consecutive patients. Pain Med 2005;6:282–6.

2. Bortsov AV, Diatchenko L, McLean SA. Complex multilocus effects of catechol-O-methyltransferase haplotypes predict pain and pain interference 6 weeks after motor vehicle collision. Neuromolecular Med 2014;16:83–93.

3. Bortsov AV, Platts-Mills TF, Peak DA, Jones JS, Swor RA, Domeier RM, Lee DC, Rathlev NK, Hendry PL, Fillingim RB, McLean SA. Pain distribution and predictors of widespread pain in the immediate aftermath of motor vehicle collision. Eur J Pain 2013;17:1243–51.

4. Bortsov AV, Platts-Mills TF, Peak DA, Jones JS, Swor RA, Domeier RM, Lee DC, Rathlev NK, Hendry PL, Fillingim RB, McLean SA. Effect of pain location and duration on life function in the year after motor vehicle collision. Pain 2014;155: 1836–45.

5. Bortsov AV, Smith JE, Diatchenko L, Soward AC, Ulirsch JC, Rossi C, Swor RA, Hauda WE, Peak DA, Jones JS, et al. Polymorphisms in the glucocorticoid receptor co-chaperone FKBP5 predict persistent musculoskeletal pain after traumatic stress exposure. Pain 2013;154:1419–26.

6. Carroll LJ, Cassidy JD, Cote P. Frequency, timing, and course of depressive symptomatology after whiplash. Spine 2006;31:E551–E556.

7. Carroll LJ, Holm LW, Hogg-Johnson S, Côté P, Cassidy JD, Haldeman S, Nordin M, Hurwitz EL, Carragee EJ, van der Velde G, et al. Course and prognostic factors for neck pain in whiplash-associated disorders (WAD): results of the Bone and Joint Decade 2000–2010 Task Force on Neck Pain and Its Associated Disorders. Spine (Phila Pa 1976) 2008;33:S83–S92.

8. Cassidy JD, Cancelliere C, Carroll LJ, Côté P, Hincapié CA, Holm LW, Hartvigsen J, Donovan J, Nygren-de Boussard C, Kristman VL, Borg J. Systematic review of self-reported prognosis in adults after mild traumatic brain injury: results of the International Collaboration on Mild Traumatic Brain Injury Prognosis. Arch Phys Med Rehabil 2014;95:S132–S151.

9. Cassidy JD, Carroll L, Cote P, Berglund A, Nygren A. Low back pain after traffic collisions: a population-based cohort study. Spine 2003;28:1002–9.

10. Castro WH. Correlation between exposure to biomechanical stress and whiplash associated disorders (WAD). Pain Res Manag 2003;8:76–8.

11. Castro WH, Meyer SJ, Becke ME, Nentwig CG, Hein MF, Ercan BI, Thomann S, Wessels U, Du Chesne AE. No stress—no whiplash? Prevalence of "whiplash" symptoms following exposure to a placebo rear-end collision. Int J Legal Med 2001;114:316–22.

12. Curatolo M, Bogduk N, Ivancic PC, McLean SA, Siegmund GP, Winkelstein BA. The role of tissue damage in whiplash-associated disorders: discussion paper 1. Spine 2011;36:S309–S315.

13. de Miguel M, Kraychete DC, Meyer Nascimento RJ. Chronic pain: cytokines, lymphocytes and chemokines. Inflamm Allergy Drug Targets 2014;13:339–49.

14. Devall AJ, Liu ZW, Lovick TA. Hyperalgesia in the setting of anxiety: sex differences and effects of the oestrous cycle in Wistar rats. Psychoneuroendocrinology 2009;34:587–96.

15. Diamond DM, Campbell AM, Park CR, Halonen J, Zoladz PR. The temporal dynamics model of emotional memory processing: a synthesis on the neurobiological basis of stress-induced amnesia, flashbulb and traumatic memories, and the Yerkes-Dodson law. Neural Plast 2007;2007:60803.

16. Do DP, Roux AVD, Hajat A, Auchincloss AH, Merkin SS, Ranjit N, Shea S, Seeman T. Circadian rhythm of cortisol and neighborhood characteristics in a population-based sample: the Multi-Ethnic Study of Atherosclerosis. Health Place 2011;17:625–32.

17. Drottning M. Acute emotional response to common whiplash predicts subsequent pain complaints: a prospective study of 107 subjects sustaining whiplash injury. Nord J Psychiatry 1995;49:293–9.

18. Ferrari R, Constantoyannis C, Papadakis N. Laypersons' expectation of the sequelae of whiplash injury: a cross-cultural comparative study between Canada and Greece. Med Sci Monit 2003;9:CR120–CR124.

19. Gay J, Abbott K. Common whiplash injury of the neck. JAMA 1953;152:1698–704.

20. Grace PM, Hutchinson MR, Maier SF, Watkins LR. Pathological pain and the neuroimmune interface. Nat Rev Immunol 2014;14:217–31.

21. Gracely RH, Lynch SA, Bennett GJ. Painful neuropathy: altered central processing maintained dynamically by peripheral input. Pain 1992;51:175–94.

22. Griggs RK, Cook J, Gargan M, Bannister G, Amirfeyz R. Mid-term follow-up of whiplash with Bournemouth Questionnaire: the significance of the initial depression to pain ratio. J Back Musculoskelet Rehabil 2014; Epub Oct 15.

23. Guy JE. The whiplash: tiny impact, tremendous injury. Ind Med Surg 1968;37:668–91.

24. Holm LW, Carroll LJ, Cassidy JD, Hogg-Johnson S, Côté P, Guzman J, Peloso P, Nordin M, Hurwitz E, van der Velde G, et al. The burden and determinants of neck pain in whiplash-associated disorders after traffic collisions: results of the Bone and Joint Decade 2000–2010 Task Force on Neck Pain and Its Associated Disorders. Spine 2008;33:S52–S59.

25. Holm LW, Carroll LJ, Cassidy JD, Skillgate E, Ahlbom A. Widespread pain following whiplash-associated disorders: incidence, course, and risk factors. J Rheumatol 2007;34:193–200.

26. Jones GT, Nicholl BI, McBeth J, Davies KA, Morriss RK, Dickens C, Macfarlane GJ. Role of road traffic accidents and other traumatic events in the onset of chronic widespread pain: results from a population-based prospective study. Arthritis Care Res (Hoboken) 2011;63:696–701.

27. Karb RA, Elliott MR, Dowd JB, Morenoff JD. Neighborhood-level stressors, social support, and diurnal patterns of cortisol: the Chicago Community Adult Health Study. Soc Sci Med 2012;75:1038–47.

28. Linnstaedt SD, Hu J, Bortsov AV, Soward AC, Swor R, Jones J, Lee D, Peak D, Domeier R, Rathlev N, et al. μ-Opioid receptor gene A118G variants and persistent pain symptoms among men and women experiencing motor vehicle collision. J Pain 2015;16(7):637–44.

29. Marcovecchio ML, Chiarelli F. The effects of acute and chronic stress on diabetes control. Sci Signal 2012;5:pt10.

30. McDonald GJ, Lord SM, Bogduk N. Long-term follow-up of patients treated with cervical radiofrequency neurotomy for chronic neck pain. Neurosurgery 1999;45:61–7; discussion 67–8.

31. McEwen BS, Eiland L, Hunter RG, Miller MM. Stress and anxiety: structural plasticity and epigenetic regulation as a consequence of stress. Neuropharmacology 2012;62:3–12.

32. McLean SA, Diatchenko L, Lee YM, Swor RA, Domeier RM, Jones JS, Jones CW, Reed C, Harris RE, Maixner W, et al. Catechol O-methyltransferase haplotype predicts immediate musculoskeletal neck pain and psychological symptoms after motor vehicle collision. J Pain 2011;12:101–7.

33. McLean SA, Ulirsch JC, Slade GD, Soward AC, Swor RA, Peak DA, Jones JS, Rathlev NK, Lee DC, Domeier RM, et al. Incidence and predictors of neck and widespread pain after motor vehicle collision among US litigants and nonlitigants. Pain 2014;155(2):309–21.

34. Merkin SS, Basurto-Davila R, Karlamangla A, Bird CE, Lurie N, Escarce J, Seeman T. Neighborhoods and cumulative biological risk profiles by race/ethnicity in a national sample of U.S. adults: NHANES III. Ann Epidemiol 2009;19:194–201.

35. Mykletun A, Glozier N, Wenzel HG, Overland S, Harvey SB, Wessely S, Hotopf M. Reverse causality in the association between whiplash and symptoms of anxiety and depression: the HUNT study. Spine 2011;36:1380–6.

36. Myrtveit SM, Skogen JC, Wenzel HG, Mykletun A. Somatic symptoms beyond those generally associated with a whiplash injury are increased in self-reported chronic whiplash. A population-based cross sectional study: the Hordaland Health Study (HUSK). BMC Psychiatry 2012;12:129.

37. Niska R, Bhuiya F, Xu J. National Hospital Ambulatory Medical Care Survey: 2007 emergency department summary. Natl Health Stat Report 2010;26:1–31.

38. Pitman RK, Rasmusson AM, Koenen KC, Shin LM, Orr SP, Gilbertson MW, Milad MR, Liberzon I. Biological studies of post-traumatic stress disorder. Nat Rev Neurosci 2012;13:769–87.

39. Qadri YJ, Bortsov AV, Orrey DC, Swor RA, Peak DA, Jones JS, Rathlev NK, Lee DC, Domeier RM, Hendry PL, Mclean SA. Genetic polymorphisms in the dopamine receptor 2 predict acute pain severity after motor vehicle collision. Clin J Pain 2014; Epub Nov 3.

40. Schutt CH, Dohan FC. Neck injury to women in auto accidents. A metropolitan plague. JAMA 1968;206:2689–92.

41. Seeman T, Epel E, Gruenewald T, Karlamangla A, McEwen BS. Socio-economic differentials in peripheral biology: cumulative allostatic load. Ann N Y Acad Sci 2010;1186:223–39.

42. Spitzer WO, Skovron ML, Salmi LR, Cassidy JD, Duranceau J, Suissa S, Zeiss E. Scientific monograph of the Quebec Task Force on whiplash-associated disorders: redefining "whiplash" and its management. Spine (Phila Pa 1976) 1995;20:1S–73S.

43. Sterling M, Elliott JM, Cabot PJ. The course of serum inflammatory biomarkers following whiplash injury and their relationship to sensory and muscle measures: a longitudinal cohort study. PLoS One 2013;8:e77903.

44. Sterling M, Jull G, Vicenzino B, Kenardy J. The development of psychological changes following whiplash injury. Pain 2003;106:481–9.

45. Sterling M, Jull G, Vicenzino B, Kenardy J. Characterization of acute whiplash-associated disorders. Spine 2004;29:182–8.

46. Ulirsch JC, Ballina LE, Soward AC, Rossi C, Hauda W, Holbrook D, Wheeler R, Foley KA, Batts J, Collette R, et al. Pain and somatic symptoms are sequelae of sexual assault: results of a prospective longitudinal study. European J Pain 2014;18:559–66.

47. Ulirsch JC, Weaver MA, Bortsov AV, Soward AC, Swor RA, Peak DA, Jones JS, Rathlev NK, Lee DC, Domeier RM, et al. No man is an island: living in a disadvantaged neighborhood influences chronic pain development after motor vehicle collision. Pain 2014;155:2116–23.

48. Vileikyte L. Stress and wound healing. Clin Dermatol 2007;25:49–55.

49. Wall PD. On the relation of injury to pain. The John J. Bonica lecture. Pain 1979;6:253–64.

50. Wynne-Jones G, Jones GT, Wiles NJ, Silman AJ, Macfarlane GJ. Predicting new onset of widespread pain following a motor vehicle collision. J Rheumatol 2006;33:968–74.

51. Wynne-Jones G, Macfarlane GJ, Silman AJ, Jones GT. Does physical trauma lead to an increase in the risk of new onset widespread pain? Ann Rheum Dis 2006;65:391–3.

CHAPTER 11

A Biopsychosocial Perspective on Motor Vehicle Collisions
Beyond Forces, Flexion, and Fractures

Dennis C. Turk and James P. Robinson

O ver 6.7 million police-reported motor vehicle collisions (MVC) occur each year in the United States [40]. A significant minority of these result in deaths (approximately 42,000) and injuries (3.4 million). Although some of these injuries are relatively minor and resolve within a few days or weeks, up to 50% of those injured report ongoing symptoms at long-term follow-up [6, 29]. The most common type of injury sustained in an MVC is whiplash [44]. The term "whiplash" (WL) has been used variously to refer to a process (the head of the passenger or driver is subject to acceleration/deceleration forces that hyperextend and hyperflex the neck [22], to the resulting injury (i.e., WL), and to the syndrome of symptoms following such an injury (whiplash syndrome) [1, 37]. The Quebec Task Force on Whiplash-Associated Disorders (WADs) [53] created a grading system of WADs caused by MVCs. This distinguishes individuals with neck pain but no physical findings (Grade I) from ones with pain as well as musculoskeletal findings such as reduced cervical range of motion (Grade II), neurological injury (Grade III), or major skeletal injury such as a fracture (Grade IV). The present chapter focuses on people with Grade I or II WADs; they comprise more than 90% of all WADs [53].

Although acute WAD symptoms are distinctly unpleasant, WAD becomes an important health issue when it becomes chronic. Estimates of the percentage of people with acute WADs who go on to develop chronic symptoms range widely from 13% to 64% [1, 12, 43]. The wide variation is likely due to the method of recruiting participants in studies (e.g., emergency department, newspapers, referred to specialist), time since MVC (hours to months), and criteria used to define WADs. Once WADs become chronic, they are extremely resistant to treatment. In this chapter, we focus on biological, psychological, and social factors that lead to chronic WADs.

The data reviewed above raise a fundamental question then: Why do some people who appear to sustain relatively minor injuries recover quickly, whereas others who have been involved in what are apparently comparable MVCs and who sustain indistinguishable physical pathology develop a diverse set of chronic symptoms, most prominently pain and significant disability? A number of potential contributors to the discrepancies have been noted and investigated (see Table 11-1). Each of the contributors has its proponents and evidential base, depending on expertise, interest, and specialty of advocates for them.

BIOPSYCHOSOCIAL PERSPECTIVE

The biopsychosocial model focuses on both disease and illness, with illness being viewed as the complex interaction of biological, psychological, social, and contextual factors [19]. The model presumes some form of physical pathology, or at least physical changes in the muscles, joints, or nerves that generate sensory input transmitted to the brain. At the periphery, nociceptive fibers transmit sensations that may or may not be interpreted as "pain." Such sensations are not yet considered pain until subjected to higher order psychological and mental processing that integrates sensory information with prior learning history, appraisals, and emotional factors to create the perception of pain. Appraisal processes are central to the perception of pain. They involve the meaning that is attributed to sensations as well as an individual's expectations and beliefs about coping strategies to ameliorate the pain

TABLE 11-1 Potential Contributors to the Development of Chronic Pain and Disability among WAD Patients

Predisposing factors
- Sociodemographic factors (e.g., age, gender, education level)
- Preexisting medical conditions
- Preexisting psychological vulnerabilities

Crash-related factors
- Characteristics of the vehicle (e.g., size and weight, head rests, seat belt use)
- Characteristics of the MVC (e.g., speed, direction of impact, amount of vehicle damage, position and awareness of occupant, involvement of fatality)

Psychological factors—Emotional responses
- Initial pain and emotional distress
- Depression
- Fear
- Posttraumatic stress disorder (PTSD)
- Anger

Psychological factors—appraisals

Environmental factors
- Reinforcement by others
- Litigation/compensation

and return to normal functioning. A person may choose to ignore the pain and continue engaging in previous levels of activity such as working or household activities, or may choose to refrain from all activity and assume the sick role and accompanying disability.

Flor and Turk [19] describe multiple ways in which a person's appraisals affect his or her processing of external or internal stimuli related to the experience of stress and pain. These include increased perception, preoccupation with and overinterpretation of physical symptoms, or inadequate perception of internal stimuli such as muscle tension levels. Moreover, they suggest that the nature of the coping response—active avoidance, passive tolerance, or depressive withdrawal—may determine the type of problem that develops, as well as the course of the illness. Flor and Turk further propose that subsequent maladaptive physiological responding, such as increased and persistent sympathetic arousal and increased and persistent muscular reactivity, as well as sensitization of central structures including the cortex, may induce or exacerbate pain episodes. Thus, they suggest that learning processes in the form of respondent conditioning of fear of activity (including social, motor, and cognitive activities), social learning, and operant learning of pain behaviors make a contribution to the chronicity of pain. They also point out that the responses of a person with a painful condition will be shaped by the behaviors of significant others. These may promote either healthy or maladaptive beliefs and responses.

In the biopsychosocial model, emphasis is shifted from the pathophysiology that may have been involved in the initiation of nociception to the patient's thoughts and feelings, and conditioned responses that influence his or her subsequent behavior and pain experiences. From this perspective, assessment of, and consequently treatment of, the patient with persistent pain requires a broad strategy that examines and addresses a wide range of psychosocial and behavioral factors, in addition to, but not to the exclusion of, biomedical ones.

Fig. 11-1 presents a schematic representation of the biopsychosocial model, depicting the overlapping sets of biological, psychological,

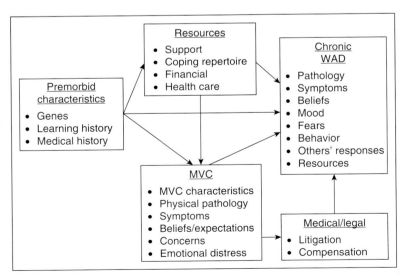

FIGURE 11-1 Biopsychosocial perspective on whiplash-associated disorders. MVC, motor vehicle collision; WAD, whiplash-associated disorder.

and social factors that affect the experience of chronic WADs, with the MVC serving as the precipitating event [see also 18, 38]. It is important to recognize that when WADs become chronic, the interplay of physical, psychosocial, behavioral, and economic factors evolves over time. Thus, none of these factors should be viewed as static.

Sociodemographic Factors

Sociodemographic factors such as sex, age, marital status, and educational levels are construed as predisposing factors in the biopsychosocial model. These factors have been studied extensively in relation to WADs. Research on the role of various sociodemographic factors has yielded inconsistent results. One recent systematic review and meta-analysis indicated that female sex and no education beyond secondary school were significant, though modest, risk factors for persistence of problems following WL injury [63]. However, another systematic review published at about the same time reported that sociodemographic factors were not related to poorer outcomes following an MVC [29]. Thus, at this point, no conclusive comments can be made as to the role of any sociodemographic variables in the development of chronicity following a WAD sustained in an MVC.

Vehicle and Crash-related Factors

Research on vehicle and crash-related factors can be conceptualized as addressing the biomechanical stimuli (e.g., loads, forces, energy) that induce WADs. Individual cohort studies have implicated a range of crash-related factors in poor recovery [47]. However, a more recent review found that the only significant vehicle or collision factor that had any significant predictive power was *not* wearing a seat belt [63], and a recent systematic review and meta-analysis concluded that crash-related (i.e., direction, speed of impact, severity of the collision) and vehicle factors (e.g., head rest, seating position, seat belt use) did not have consistent predictive value [29].

Physical Pathology

Research on structural and physiological abnormalities among WAD patients can be construed as addressing the biomechanical responses of individuals to the strains created by MVCs. Various authors have implicated a wide range of structures in the pathophysiology of WADs—including bones, facet joints, intervertebral disks, ligaments, muscles, and neural structures. Despite decades of research, it has been difficult to identify the structural or physiological abnormalities that underlie WADs. In particular, radiological studies designed to identify structural abnormalities in WAD patients have generally failed to do so [6]. The disappointing results of radiological studies have led some investigators to assert that in more than 90% of WL claims, no organic pathology can be detected [17].

In interpreting studies on the structural/physiological substrates of WAD, several issues need to be considered. First, although it is logical to assume that radiological studies should be able to detect structural abnormalities created by the forces generated during MVCs, and that such abnormalities should permit pathoanatomic diagnoses to be given to WAD patients, some investigators reject the primacy of imaging studies in the diagnosis of these patients. In particular, Lord and colleagues [33, 34] have asserted that responses of patients to local anesthetic blocks represent the best method of diagnosing structural/physiological abnormalities. On the basis of patients' responses to local anesthetic blocks and subsequent facet neurotomies, these and other investigators have concluded that a substantial proportion of WAD patients have abnormalities in their cervical facet joints [34, 35]. For purposes of this chapter, the broad point is that statements about the frequency of biological abnormalities in WAD patients are uninterpretable unless there is agreement on the criteria for diagnosing these abnormalities.

Another problem is that research on the structural basis of WAD assumes that a pain generator in the cervical spine (e.g., an inflamed facet joint) leads in a straightforward way to WAD symptoms. Thus, it is assumed that the nervous system of a WAD patient responds to tissue damage in an uncomplicated way, and is "veridical" in the sense that the pain experiences of a patient accurately reflect this damage [49]. This assumption is challenged by a growing body of research indicating that persistent WAD is often mediated by sensitization of the central nervous system [11, 28, 61]. As an example of problems in this area, Turk et al. [60] found that 46% of a cohort of people with WADs with no known other injuries met the tender point criterion for a diagnosis of fibromyalgia—they reported tenderness in at least 11 of the 18 sites designated by the American College of Rheumatology for the diagnosis [65]. The significance of this widespread hyperalgesia is not entirely clear, but it certainly suggests that the pain experienced by many people with WADs is not reducible to a single structural abnormality. To the extent that persistent WAD pain is mediated by altered nervous system responsivity rather than by ongoing nociceptive input from the neck, there is no reason to expect a one-to-one relation between WAD symptoms and a definable structural lesion in the neck.

A third issue is that even when diagnoses of structural pathology in the cervical spines of WAD patients can be made, the diagnoses are qualitative and thus do not provide insight into why some WAD patients report prolonged pain and demonstrate severe disability, whereas others complain of only mild, transitory symptoms.

Finally, attempts to identify the structural basis of WAD must be tempered by the difficulties that physicians and researchers have repeatedly encountered when they have attempted to pinpoint the pain generator underlying axial pain in any portion of the spine [2, 16, 27, 32].

Premorbid Psychological Characteristics

As early as 1953, Gay and Abbot [22] mentioned "neurotic reactions" in WL, noting that particular psychological factors *predisposed* an individual to chronic problems after an accident. In 1971, Hodge [25] stated that patients with chronic symptoms after MVC have preexisting psychopathology and that the collision offers a solution for their preexisting neurosis. It seems reasonable that preexisting psychological status may predispose *some* individuals to chronic emotional disturbances following MVC. However, it is difficult to identify such predisposing psychological factors, at least partly because information about the pre-accident psychological functioning of individuals with WL is often not available.

Initial Psychological Responses to MVC

Research has generally indicated just after a WL injury that the severity of individuals' pain and the intensity of their emotional reactions have implications for the clinical course that they are likely to follow [9, 29, 48, 52, 63]. Patients who rate their pain intensity as very high have been found to be at risk for persistent WAD (although this relationship has not always been found) [5]. Initial emotional reaction to the accident, rather than preexisting psychological status, has been shown to predict chronicity [13, 21]. For example, acute emotional distress has been shown to be related to pain severity 1 month following an MVC [36].

Postcollision Psychological Factors—Anxiety and Depression

Psychological symptoms following a MVC have been thoroughly documented. Jaspers [26] reviewed the literature on psychological symptoms after MVCs and reported that psychological sequelae of such accidents include anxiety and mood disorders. Anxiety and depression are observed in 10% of post-MVC people, and an additional 10% continue to have posttraumatic stress symptoms 1 year after the accident [36]. Disabling emotional symptoms have been observed in as many as 33% of people post-MVA up to 2 years after the accident [21]. In a large study, Wenzel et al. [64] found an association among anxiety, depression, and pain and disability in people with histories of MVCs more than 2 years prior to the assessment but not in those with acute injuries, suggesting that symptom persistence is the instigator for emotional distress.

A population-based study of over 5000 individuals who made insurance claims or who were seeking health care following WADs post-MVC found that 42.3% developed depressive symptoms within 6 weeks of the crash and these symptoms were recurrent or persisted in 37.6% [5]. Importantly, preinjury mental health problems increased the risk of later onset of depressive symptoms and maintenance of symptoms up to 12 months postcollision. However, more than 40% of the sample with no prior mental health problems developed depressive symptoms within 6 weeks of the MVC, and another 18% during the year following the MVC.

In contrast, Radanov et al. [45, 46] reported no elevations in depression scores among people with WADs at any point following the collision regardless of recovery status. These inconsistencies likely reflect differences in selection criteria (treatment seeking, insurance claimants, emotional symptoms vs. psychiatric diagnosis), sample characteristics, methods of assessing emotional distress, and frequency and methods used to obtain follow-up data. The thrust of research supports the conclusion that preexisting psychological disturbances, immediate emotional reaction, coupled with medical complications, contribute to chronicity of WADs at least for some people [36].

Posttraumatic Stress Disorder (PTSD)

PTSD would seem to be particularly relevant given the trauma sustained in an MVC. Symptoms of PTSD (e.g., spontaneous and unwanted flashback memories) have been found in a proportion (up to 25% [26]) of people following a WL injury due to an MVC [30], and these symptoms have shown prognostic capacity for poor functional recovery [55]. (PTSD in WADs patients is discussed in more detail in the chapters by Sullivan and Sterling in this volume).

Fear and Avoidance

Investigators have proposed a fear-avoidance model to incorporate the role of catastrophizing and negative symptom beliefs in illness behavior [62]. According to this model, fearful people often engage in behaviors designed to escape or avoid negative stimuli, and become hypervigilant to stimuli associated with the feared situation. Many patients with chronic pain, especially those who attribute their symptoms to traumas such as MVCs, are fearful of engaging in activities that they believe may either contribute to further injury or exacerbate their symptoms [29, 50]. Avoidance of activities may, in the short term, lead to symptom reduction, but, over time, restriction of activities is likely to lead to decreased functional capacities as a result of deconditioning. Also, avoidance of activity has the unfortunate consequence of preventing corrective feedback. Health care providers may inadvertently contribute to avoidance of activity by ordering sophisticated diagnostic tests in search of occult physical pathology, providing patients with cervical collars that restrict neck movements and advising them to avoid activities that hurt. These activities and messages contribute to the patient's anxiety that "hurt equals harm" and that something is seriously wrong with their bodies.

Hypervigilance for symptoms represents an attentional bias that many people with WADs exhibit. An attentional bias is a selective attention toward specific information, most often in relation to threatening information. People who experience recurrent symptoms may develop a pattern of behavior in which they are constantly on high alert for future pain. This hypervigilance may lead patients to avoid activity altogether or to stop activity at the first sign of symptoms. Hypervigilance for pain has been associated with increased pain intensity, disability, and pain-related health care utilization in a variety of populations of patients with chronic pain [10]. It is important to bear in mind that for the individual with the symptoms, being hypervigilant to pain makes perfect sense—paying attention to a potential threat is an important survival mechanism. Although this is true in the short term, hypervigilance in the context of chronic WAD can lead to excessive activity avoidance and fear. To promote a healthy amount of attention to symptoms, WADs patients may require ongoing education about the difference between monitoring symptoms and excessive focus on symptoms.

Results of studies on the predictive ability of the fear-avoidance model in WAD are not consistent. Whereas Nederhand et al. [41] and Nieto et al. [42] reported that patients with greater levels of pain-related fear were more likely to develop chronic WAD-related disability fear, Sterling et al. [54] found no significant relationship between pain-related fear and the development of chronic pain and disability after an MVC.

Anger and Perceived Injustice

The emotional reactions of individuals with WADs include anger as well as depression and fear. WADs patients may experience anger directed toward the individual who caused the crash, the health care providers for not alleviating persistent symptoms, third-party payers who they feel do not believe them, family members, and even themselves for contributing to the circumstances surround the MVC. Sullivan et al. [58] have characterized this as "perceived injustice" in relation to pain that they define as an appraisal reflecting the severity and irreparability of pain-related loss, blame, and unfairness. They found that perceived injustice was a significant predictor of prolonged work absence [56] and predicted persistent symptoms of posttraumatic stress [58] following a WL injury.

Appraisals and Beliefs

The ways in which people respond to psychological and physical insults depend not only on their emotional reactions to the injurious stimuli, but also on their beliefs and appraisals regarding the stimuli. The significance of these cognitive processes has been examined in research on WAD [3, 4, 50]. It should be noted at the outset that beliefs and appraisals regarding threatening stimuli are by no means entirely separate from emotional reactions to the stimuli. In fact, there are complex interplays between people's emotional reactions and their beliefs and appraisals. Thus, for example, the researchers who developed the fear-avoidance model emphasize that people's appraisals of their painful condition often set the stage for the development of fear.

Several studies have implicated the role of the patient's idiosyncratic appraisals of his or her symptoms, expectations regarding the cause of the symptoms, and the meaning of the symptoms as essential in understanding the individual's report of pain and the maintenance of subsequent disability associated with chronic WAD [3, 57, 59]. A recent meta-analysis [31] reported that among people with low back pain and neck pain, appraisals regarding self-efficacy, along with fear and psychological distress, significantly mediated the relationship between pain and disability.

Social and Environmental Factors

Reinforcement by Others

The experience of pain is largely private, highly personal, and subjective. However, there are social features associated with pain. People with chronic pain do not exist in a vacuum—they are partners, employees, and friends. That is, they are an integral part of many complex socioenvironmental systems. Patients display a broad range of responses that communicate to others that they are experiencing pain, distress, and suffering—"pain behaviors." Pain behaviors include verbal reports, paralinguistic vocalizations (e.g., sighs, moans), motor activity, facial expressions, body postures and gesturing (e.g., rubbing a painful body part, grimacing), functional limitations (reclining for extensive periods), and behaviors designed to reduce pain (e.g., taking medication). Although there is no one-to-one relationship between these pain behaviors and self-report of pain, they are at least modestly correlated. The fact that behaviors are observable is important as they may elicit responses from significant others including health care providers. The nature of the responses may reinforce the behaviors positively, thereby increasing the likelihood that they will be maintained. Conversely, the behaviors may be negatively reinforced or even punished, in which case the probability of their occurrence will likely be reduced. It is important to emphasize that behavioral changes among WADs patients in response to environmental reinforcement are often brought about through conditioning, and thus are not necessarily consciously motivated.

Litigation and Compensation

There is a large literature on the effect of litigation and attorney involvement on outcomes of WAD [7, 8, 20, 39, 51]. Results have been inconsistent. For example, whereas several studies reported a negative effect of attorney involvement and litigation on recovery from WAD [14, 23], others [24] did not find such an effect. It is beyond the scope of this chapter to review this often contentious literature on the effect of litigation and attorney involvement on outcomes of WAD. Our interpretation of this literature is that it does, on balance, support the hypothesis that attorney involvement, participation in litigation, or both is a negative prognostic factor for individuals with WAD.

CONCLUSIONS

Overall, research evaluating factors predictive of chronicity in WAD symptoms has yielded equivocal results. Although some investigators have asserted that psychological factors are more relevant than collision severity in predicting both duration and severity of symptoms in Grade 1 and 2 WADs [48], the most parsimonious conclusion from research in this area is that essentially all the hypothesized contributors to chronicity have either failed to demonstrate predictive validity or have demonstrated only modest associations with outcomes of WAD (outlined in Table 11-1). Furthermore, current management strategies, which are presumably informed by research on factors contributing to chronicity, do not appear to have lessened the incidence of the transition from acute to chronic state [15].

Emerging evidence suggests that a biopsychosocial perspective that considers premorbid history, resources available (i.e., personal, social, health care, financial) at the onset of a WAD, biomechanical features associated with a collision, pathophysiology, initial symptoms, individuals' beliefs and expectations, and medical-legal factors offers the most promising approach to the prediction of poor outcome following MVC. Thus, better understanding and treatment of patients with WADs will need to be based on an integrated biopsychosocial perspective in contrast to relying on any individual set of prognostic factors.

REFERENCES

1. Barnsley L, Lord S, Bogduk N. Whiplash injury. Pain 1994;58:283–307.

2. Borenstein DG, O'Mara JW Jr, Boden SD, Lauerman WC, Jacobson A, Platenberg C, Schellinger D, Wiesel SW. The value of magnetic resonance imaging of the lumbar spine to predict low-back pain in asymptomatic subjects: a seven-year follow-up study. J Bone Joint Surg Am 2001;83:1306–11.

3. Bostick GP, Carroll LJ, Brown CA, Harley D, Gross DP. Predictive capacity of pain beliefs and catastrophizing in whiplash associatd disorders. Injury 2013;44:1465–71.

4. Buitenhuis J, de Jong PJ, Jaspers JP, Groothoff JW. Catastrophizing and causal beliefs in whiplash. Spine 2008;33:2427–33.

5. Carroll LJ, Cassidy JD, Cote P. Frequency, timing, and course of depressive symptomatology after whiplash. Spine 2006;16:E551–E556.

6. Carroll LJ, Holm LW, Hogg-Johnson S, Côté P, Cassidy JD, Haldeman S, Nordin M, Hurwitz EL, Carragee EJ, van der Velde G, et al. Course and prognostic factors for neck pain in whiplash-associated-disorders (WAD): results of the Bone and Joint Decade 2000–2010 Task Force on Neck Pain and Its Associated Disorders. Spine (Phila Pa 1976) 2008;33:S83–S92.

7. Cassidy JD, Carroll LJ, Cote P, Lemstra M, Berglund A, Nygren A. Effect of eliminating compensation for pain and suffering on the outcome of insurance claims for whiplash injury. N Engl J Med 2000;342:1179–86.

8. Clionsky M. Effect of eliminating compensation for pain and suffering on the outcome of insurance claims. N Engl J Med 2000;343:1119.

9. Cote P, Hogg-Johnson S, Cassidy JD, Carroll L, Frank JW. The association between neck pain intensity, physical functioning, depressive symptomatology and time-to-claim-closure after whiplash. J Clin Epidemiol 2001;54:275–86.

10. Crombez G, van Damme S, Eccleston C. Hypervigilance to pain: an experimental and clinical analysis. Pain 2005;116:4–7.

11. Curatolo M, Arendt-Nielsen L, Petersen-Felix S. Evidence, mechanisms, and clinical implications of central hypersensitivity in chronic pain after whiplash injury. Clin J Pain 2004;20:469–76.

12. Deans GT, Magalliard JN, Kerr M, Rutherford WH. Neck sprain—a major cause of disability following car accidents. Injury 1987;18:10–12.

13. Drottning M, Staff PH, Levin L, Malt UF. Acute emotional response to common whiplash predicts subsequent pain complaints—a prospective study of 107 subjects sustaining whiplash injury. Nordic J Psychiat 1995;49:293–300.

14. Dufton JA, Kopec JA, Wong H, Cassidy JD, Quon J, McIntosh G, Koehoorn M. Prognostic factors associated with minimal improvement following acute whiplash-associated disorders. Spine 2006;31:E759–65; discussion E766.

15. Elliott JM, Noteboom JTR, Flynn TW, Sterling M. Characterization of acute and chronic whiplash-associated disorders. J Orthop Sports Phys Ther 2009;39:312–23.

16. Englund M, Guermazi A, Gale D, Hunter DJ, Aliabadi P, Clancy M, Felson DT. Incidental meniscal findings on knee MRI in middle-aged and elderly persons. N Engl J Med 2008;359:1108–15.

17. Ferrari R, Russell AS, Carroll LJ, Cassidy JD. A re-examination of the whiplash-associated disorders (WAD) as a systemic illness. Ann Rheum Dis 2005;64:1337–42.

18. Ferrari R, Schrader H. The late whiplash syndrome: a biopsychosocial approach. J Neurol Neurosurg Psychiat 2001;70:722–6.

19. Flor H, Turk DC. Chronic pain: an integrated biobehavioral perspective. Seattle, WA: International Association for the Study of Pain Press; 2011.

20. Freeman MD, Rossignol AM. Effect of eliminating compensation for pain and suffering on the outcome of insurance claims. N Engl J Med 2000;343:1118–9.

21. Gargan M, Bannister G, Main C, Hollis S. The behavioral response to whiplash injury. J Bone Joint Surg Br 1997;79:523–6.

22. Gay J, Abbot K. Common whiplash injuries of the neck. J Am Med Assoc 1953;152:1698–704.

23. Gun RT, Osti OL, O'Riordan A, Mpelasoka F, Eckerwall CG, Smyth JF. Risk factors for prolonged disability after whiplash injury: a prospective study. Spine 2005;30:386–91.

24. Hendricks EJ, Scholten-Peeters GG, van der Windt DA, Neeleman-van der Steen CW, Oostendorp RA, Verhagen AP. Prognostic factors for poor recovery in acute whiplash patients. Pain 2005;114:408–16.

25. Hodge JR. The whiplash neurosis. Psychosomatics 1971;12:245–9.

26. Jaspers JPC. Whiplash and post-traumatic stress disorder. Disabil Rehabil 1998;20: 397–404.

27. Jensen MC, Brant-Zawadski MN, Obuchowski N, Modic MT, Malkasian D, Ross JS. Magnetic resonance imaging of the lumbar spine in people with back pain. N Engl J Med 1994;331:69–73.

28. Ji RR, Kohno T, Moore KA, Woolf CJ. Central sensitization and LTP: do pain and memory share similar mechanisms? Trends Neurosci 2003;26:696–705.

29. Kamper SJ, Rebbeck TJ, Maher CC, McAuley JH, Sterling M. Course and prognostic factors of whiplash: a systematic review and meta-analysis. Pain 2008;136:617–29.

30. Kongsted A, Bendix T, Qerama E, Kasch H, Bach KW, Korsholm L, Jensen TS. Acute stress response and recovery after whiplash injuries. A one-year prospective study. Eur J Pain 2008;12:455–63.

31. Lee H, Hubscher M, Moseley GL, Kamper SJ, Traeger AC, Mansellf G, McAuley JH. How does pain lead to disability? A systematic review and meta-analysis of mediation studies in people with back and neck pain. Pain 2015;156:988–97.

32. Link TM, Steinbach LS, Ghosh S, Ries M, Lu Y, Lane N, Majumdar S. Osteoarthritis: MR imaging findings in different stages of disease and correlation with clinical findings. Radiology 2003;226:373–81.

33. Lord S, Barnsley L, Wallis BJ, Bogduk N. Chronic cervical zygapophyseal joint pain after whiplash: a placebo-controlled prevalence study. Spine 1996;21:1737–45.

34. Lord SM, Barnsley L, Wallis BJ, McDonald GJ, Bogduk N. Percutaneous radio-frequency neurotomy for chronic zygapophysial-joint pain. N Engl J Med 1996;335:1721–6.

35. Manchikanti L, Singh V, Rivera J, Pampati V. Prevalence of cervical facet joint pain in chronic neck pain. Pain Physician 2002;5:243–9.

36. Mayou R, Bryant B, Duthie R. Psychiatric consequences of road traffic accidents. BMJ 1993;307:647–51.

37. Mayou R, Radanov BP. Whiplash neck injury. J Psychosom Res 1996;40:461–74.

38. McLean SA, Clauw DJ, Abelson JL, Liberzon I. The development of persistent pain and psychological morbidity after motor vehicle collision: integrating the potential role of stress response systems into a biopsychosocial model. Psychosom Med 2005;67:783–90.

39. Merskey H, Teasell RW. Effect of eliminating compensation for pain and suffering on the outcome of insurance claims. N Engl J Med 2000;343:1119.

40. National Highway Traffic Safety Administration. Traffic Safety Facts 1997. A compilation of motor vehicle crash data from the Fatality Analysis Reporting System and the general estimates system. Washington, DC: U.S. Department of Transportation; 1998.

41. Nederhand MJ, Ijzerman MJ, Hermens HJ, Turk DC, Zilvold G. Predictive value of fear avoidance in developing chronic neck pain disability: consequences for clinical decision making. Arch Phys Med Rehabil 2004;85:496–501.

42. Nieto R, Miro J, Huguet A. The fear-avoidance model in whiplash injuries. Eur J Pain 2009;13:518–23.

43. Pennie B, Agambar L. Patterns of injury and recovery in whiplash. Injury 1991;22:57–9.

44. Quinlan KP, Annest JL, Myers B, Rayan G, Hill H. Neck strains and sprains among motor vehicle occupants—United States, 2000. Accid Anal Prev 2000;36:21–7.

45. Radanov B, Berge S, Sturzenegger M, Augusting KF. Course of psychological variables in whiplash injury: a 2-year follow-up with age, gender and education-matched patients. Pain 1996;64:429–34.

46. Radanov B, Di Stefano G, Schnidrig A, Sturzeneggar M. Psychosocial stress, cognitive performance, and disability after common whiplash. J Psychosom Res 1993;37:1–10.

47. Radanov B, Sturzeneggar M, di Stefano G, Schnidrig A. Relationship between early somatic, radiological, cognitive, and psychosocial findings and outcome during a one-year follow-up in 117 patients suffering from chronic whiplash. Br J Rheumatol 1994;64:442–8.

48. Richter M, Ferrari R, Otte D, Kuensbeck HW, Blauth M, Krettek C. Correlation of clinical findings, collision parameters, and psychological factors in the outcome of whiplash associated disorders. J Neurol Neurosurg Psychiatry 2004;745:758–64.

49. Robinson JP, Apkarian AV. Low back pain. In: Mayer EA, Bushnell MC, editors. Functional pain syndromes: presentation and pathophysiology. Seattle, WA: International Association for the Study of Pain Press; 2009. pp. 23–53.

50. Robinson JP, Theodore BR, Dansie EJ, Wilson HD, Turk DC. The role of fear of movement in subacute whiplash-associated disorders grades I and II with fear of activity. Pain 2013;154:393–401.

51. Russell RS. Effect of eliminating compensation for pain and suffering on the outcome of insurance claims. N Engl J Med 2000;343:1119–20.

52. Scholten-Peeters GG, Verhagen AP, Bekkering GE, van der Windt DA, Barnsley L, Oostendorp RA, Hendriks EJ. Prognostic factors of whiplash-associated disorders: a systematic review of prospective cohort studies. Pain 2003;104:303–22.

53. Spitzer WO, Skovron ML, Salmi LR, Cassidy JD, Duranceau J, Suissa S, Zeiss E. Scientific monograph of the Quebec Task Force on whiplash-associated disorders: redefining "whiplash" and its management. Spine 1995;20(8, Suppl):1S–73S.

54. Sterling M, Jull G, Vicenzino B, Kenardy J. Sensory hypersensitivity occurs soon after whiplash injury and is associated with poor recovery. Pain 2003;104:509–17.

55. Sterling M, Jull G, Vicenzino B, Kenardy J, Darnell R. Physical and psychological factors predict outcome following whiplash injury. Pain 2005;114:141–8.

56. Sullivan MJ, Adams H, Horan S, Mahar D, Boland D, Gross R. The role of perceived injustice in the experience of chronic pain and disability: scale development and validation. J Occup Rehabil 2008;18:249–61.

57. Sullivan MJ, Adams H, Martel MO, Scott W, Wideman T. Catastrophizing and perceived injustice: risk factors for the transition to chronicity after whiplash injury. Spine 2011;36:5244–9.

58. Sullivan M, Thibault P, Simmonds M, Milioto M, Cantin AP, Velly A. Pain, perceived injustice and the persistence of post-traumatic stress symptoms during the course of rehabilitation for whiplash injuries. Pain 2009;145:325–31.

59. Thompson DP, Oldham JA, Urmston M, Woby SR. Cognitive determinants of pain and disability in patients with chronic whiplash-associated disorders: a cross-sectional observational study. Physiotherapy 2010;96:151–9.

60. Turk DC, Robinson JP, Burwinkle T. Prevalence of fibromyalgia tender points following whiplash injury. J Pain 2006;7(Suppl 2):S27.

61. Van Oosterwijck J, Nijs J, Meeus M, Paul L. Evidence for central sensitization in chronic whiplash: a systematic literature review. Eur J Pain 2013;17:299–312.

62. Vlaeyen JW, Kole-Snijders AM, Rotteveel AM, Ruesink R, Heuts PH. The role of fear of movement/(re)injury in pain disability. J Occup Rehabil 1995;5:235–52.

63. Walton DM, Pretty J, MacDermid JC, Teasell RW. Risk factors for persistent problems following whiplash injury. Results of a systematic review and meta-analysis. J Orthop Sports Phys Ther 2009;39:334–50.

64. Wenzel H, Gro H, Tangen T, Mykletun A, Dahl AA. A population study of anxiety and depression among person who report whiplash traumas. J Psyhosom Res 2002;53:831–5.

65. Wolfe F, Smythe HA, Yunus MB, Bennett RM, Bombardier C, Goldenberg DL, Tugwell P, Campbell SM, Abeles M, Clark P, et al. The American College of Rheumatology 1990 Criteria for the Classification of Fibromyalgia. Report of the Multicenter Criteria Committee. Arthritis Rheum 1990;33:160–72.

CHAPTER 12

Improving Psychologically Oriented Treatments for WAD

Steven James Linton

For reasons not fully understood, many patients who sustain a WAD (whiplash-associated disorder) recover quickly, while others develop long-term problems. Psychological factors offer one enticing explanation for why WAD may become persistent [25], and psychologically oriented treatments have therefore been evaluated in some intervention studies. Indeed, because WAD all too often develops into a debilitating problem, it presents a unique challenge for the application of psychologically oriented pain interventions. Indeed, psychological treatments have been proposed as a way of implementing a biopsychosocial approach to a difficult problem [19] (see Turk and Robinson Chapter 11 in this volume for an overview of the biopsychosocial model in WAD). Yet the application of psychological treatments is not uniform, and they are offered at different points in time, in diverse formats, by a range of professionals, in a wide variety of settings. Consequently, there is a need to sort out what psychological treatment components might be applicable, how well they work, and for whom. Since WAD continues to be a problem for the individual, their family, the workplace, and society, there is also a need to examine how psychological approaches might be improved.

My point of departure, then, is how psychology might contribute to meeting the challenge of effectively treating WAD. To this end, the aim of my chapter is to review, with an eye on improvement, the role of psychological treatments for WAD. I will first provide important background for understanding what psychological interventions may be applicable and when they might best be applied. Subsequently, I will examine some of the treatments themselves and explore the results obtained to date. This is central since the field is facing major challenges in providing effective interventions that will prevent chronic WAD, rehabilitate those with persistent WAD, while at the same time being cost-effective and applicable to several clinical settings. Finally, given this great challenge, I will emphasize some ways in which the application of psychological interventions might be improved.

SALIENT PSYCHOLOGICAL FEATURES

Psychological interventions target certain underlying psychological mechanisms that are believed to be of the greatest importance. While many individual variables have been implicated, let us focus on a few of the most fundamental factors. To understand how psychological factors impact on people suffering WAD, it is crucial to underscore how the problem develops or remits over time. As with other forms of pain, WAD is triggered by an injury, and there are several ensuing trajectories for recovery (full or partial) or development toward persistence (recurrent problem, stepped problem) [8, 32]. A particular feature of this process is that the repeated episodes of pain provide plenty of opportunity for psychological factors to impact upon the course of development [26, 53]. I suspect that this occurs in stages where certain factors like fear, catastrophizing (the tendency to misinterpret and exaggerate situations as dangerous), and symptoms of PTSD are prevalent early on. As time goes on without recovery, other processes are added such as worry, frustration, and difficulties in problem solving caused by persistent pain. In the chronic stage, individuals with WAD are plagued by a host of psychological factors that maintain the problem (e.g., depression, inactivity, inflexibility, shame, guilt [28]).

Table 12-1 provides an overview of some basic psychological factors that may influence the course of WAD and suggested time points for their peak relevance. The table also shows some suggested treatments

TABLE 12-1	Examples of Psychological Factors that Affect WAD According to the Time Point for Their Peak Relevance	
Time Point	*Psychological Factor(s)*	*Targeted Intervention Strategy*
Injury	Posttraumatic Stress Disorder symptoms	Trauma-focused CBT for PTSD
Early (acute)	Fear and avoidance including catastrophic worry	CBT targeting PTSD, fear avoidance, (e.g., exposure).
Recurrent episodes	Increasing worry, frustration, distress, goal conflict, decreasing function, and flexibility	Multimodal CBT pain interventions. Exposure for fear avoidance.
Persistent (chronic)	Depression, disability, inflexibility, multiple symptoms	Multimodal CBT chronic pain rehabilitation interventions. Hybrid CBT targeting emotion, avoidance and pain.

targeting the psychological factor noted and these listed will be examined more closely below. As Table 12-1 shows, several psychological factors on the behavioral, cognitive, and emotional planes come into play. Typically, WAD is associated with a traumatic injury (e.g., an automobile accident), and early research demonstrated a link between the injury and problems associated with Posttraumatic Stress Disorder (PTSD) [7]. The injury also triggers pain and soft-tissue symptoms like swelling and stiffness. The Fear and Avoidance model is therefore particularly applicable during the early stage of the problem [58, 59]. Briefly, this model suggests that the pain triggers catastrophic thoughts and fear that focus attention on the injury and result in the avoidance of movements believed to be dangerous for exacerbating the pain and causing further injury. When the problem recurs or persists, this is thought to trigger more catastrophic worry, and a host of negative emotions including anger and frustration [14, 52]. The emotional distress and cognitive activity is believed to contribute to the problem and makes solutions more difficult. Anger, for example, is a prevalent reaction known to be related to chronic pain [52]. Further, some patients may feel victimized since the accident was not their fault and they may have experienced problems in receiving adequate treatment [48]. Increasingly, they may face important goal conflicts (e.g., on the one hand wanting to participate in work, family, and social activities, while at the same time not wanting to exacerbate their pain or the injury) [56]. This process may result in even more distress including shame and guilt, inflexible thinking patterns that make creative problem solving difficult and generally leave the individual vulnerable to a variety of additional problems such as unemployment, relational problems, and depression [28]. This range of factors opens the door to a range of treatment interventions that might be initiated from the point of injury forward.

Psychological Interventions and Their Effectiveness

Psychological interventions are designed to target various underlying mechanisms, and they are often provided in a diversity of settings, from emergency rooms to rehabilitation clinics. The amount of intervention provided also varies grossly, with some programs offering only an hour or 2 as part of a broader treatment, while others provide considerable amounts. Typically, psychological interventions are coordinated with other interventions, and they may be provided by psychologists or sometimes by other members of a team. Thus, psychological treatments are quite heterogeneous, and this variation may account for differences in outcome in addition to the actual choice of the psychological treatment.

PTSD-Focused Treatments

Many people sustain a WAD in a motor vehicle collision that may also trigger PTSD symptoms [47]. It is estimated that at least 25% of those with WAD associated with a car crash also display significant PTSD symptoms [47]. This anxiety disorder comprises three groups of symptoms: avoidance of stimuli associated with the accident, arousal (e.g., hypervigilance and the re-experiencing of the trauma). In addition to the disability itself, pain catastrophizing and perceived injustice have been found to be salient factors propelling the problem Sullivan et al. [50]. Fortunately, cognitive-behavioral therapy (CBT) has shown clear benefit for PTSD-associated problems with large effect sizes [3, 6]. One central theme in these treatments is to focus on the trauma. In particular, exposure training (similar to that used for phobias) is employed where patients are gradually exposed until habituation occurs for the stimuli that trigger the symptoms. For those patients with a WAD diagnosis who also have PTSD, psychological treatment may offer clear help.

As an example, a randomized controlled trial compared a trauma-focused CBT intervention with a waiting-list control for those with chronic (Mean = 28 months) WAD (grades II and III) and comorbid PTSD [11]. The treatment was based on guidelines for PTSD interventions and consisted of 10, 1-hour individual sessions with a psychologist. The results, despite a relatively small number of participants (13 per group), showed large and significant differences. In terms of the PTSD, those in the CBT group experienced a significant reduction of symptoms, and 8 of 13 no longer fulfilled the criteria for the disorder. Moreover, the CBT group, relative to the control, also had large improvements in a variety of other variables including function. Clinically significant reductions in both the PTSD and the WAD symptoms underscore the potential of this type of treatment. Targeting of treatment to those with clear psychological problems may be appropriate since the content, duration, and delivery of psychological treatment to all individuals with WAD have limitations. For example, the inclusion of psychological treatment as an add-on to physical therapy has not shown effectiveness [19, 45], and some individuals do not accept such treatments [16, 24]. Thus, targeting PTSD symptoms with an evidence-based CBT intervention has promise for those suffering comorbid problems.

Fear Avoidance Targeted

A second target for psychological treatment is based on the fear and avoidance conceptualization described above [41, 58]. In order to treat the avoidance behavior and relieve catastrophic worry and fear, exposure in vivo is recommended since it has a good evidence base for chronic pain in general [2, 36, 60]. Indeed, patients with a WAD diagnosis often avoid movements they believe will exacerbate their pain or result in injury. Treatment is based on identifying movements that provoke this fear and therefore maintain avoidance, and then systematically exposing the patient to these movements to achieve extinction of the feared response.

Several investigations have shown that exposure may be helpful for those fulfilling the criteria for fear and avoidance. First, a controlled trial with 8 patients demonstrated that exposure was viable and resulted in a larger decrease in fear, pain intensity, and disability than that in a comparison group receiving activity training [10]. Second, a randomized controlled trial featuring exposure and acceptance demonstrated that a 10-session protocol resulted in significantly larger improvements in disability, satisfaction, fear, and depression relative to a waiting-list control [62]. Although participants had symptoms for an average of nearly 7 years, this relatively brief treatment had a substantial effect.

A well-designed and executed trial featured the role of fear in the treatment of WAD [41]. This study of nearly 200 people with relatively minor WAD symptoms (grades I and II [46]) for 3 months compared three types of intervention: an information booklet, the booklet plus didactic discussions, and exposure therapy. Treatment was brief, just 3, 2-hour sessions. However, based on pre- to posttreatment evaluations, the exposure treatment resulted in superior outcomes (e.g., for pain intensity and neck function). Indeed, on the Neck Disability Index [57], those receiving exposure improved nearly 15 points, on average, which is far better than the minimally clinically important level that has been found to range between 3.5 and 9.5 points [41]. Importantly, this study also showed that a reduction in fear was the most important predictor of improvements in function. Thus, this study provides strong support for the idea that fear and avoidance is an important factor and that successfully treating it leads to clinically notable improvements.

Early Prevention

Because psychological factors are key drivers in the development of persistent chronic WAD, early psychological interventions might prevent chronicity. About 50% of those with WAD will report neck pain

1 year after the injury, and the main prognostic factors include passive coping, depression, and fear of movement [8]. Moreover, the outcome of rehabilitation efforts is directly related to the duration of the problem. For instance, a comparison of patients with three different durations of WAD receiving the same 10-week rehabilitation intervention showed drastic differences [1]. While 80% of those with subacute WAD (4–12 weeks) returned to work after the intervention, only 32% of those entering the program with chronic WAD (6–18 months) returned to work [1]. This suggests that early interventions may be highly effective.

In an attempt to provide an early intervention for WAD, an initial program offered 10, 1-hour sessions of graded activity as an add-on to usual physical therapy [49]. Thus, this program targeted activity levels using activity logs, scheduling, and graded activity rather than PTSD or fear avoidance. Although the study did not employ a randomized design, a control group consisted of similar patients who received physical therapy. Four weeks after completion of the interventions, 75% of those in the physical therapy and activity training group returned to work as opposed to 50% of those receiving the usual physical therapy.

Another approach to prevention has been to provide treatment soon after injury. The PTSD symptoms associated with an injury are a target since the literature on PTSD shows that individually delivered, multiple sessions of CBT including exposure techniques for patients with severe symptoms are effective in the first weeks [24]. However, since psychological symptoms associated with an injury normally diminish with time, caution has also been warranted since ill-reasoned early interventions may actually interfere with this natural recovery process. For example, various forms of discussion groups and so-called "debriefing" have been employed in the aftermath of significant traumas, but reviews of the literature suggest that they lead to an *increase* in the rate of developing PTSD [24, 42].

A recent investigation examined whether providing early treatments including psychological methods would be effective in reducing the rate of developing chronicity [22]. Over 100 patients with WAD, grade II, of less than 4 weeks' duration were randomly assigned to usual care or a multiprofessional management protocol. The multiprofessional protocol included the possibility to receive medical (including analgesics), physical therapy (including exercise), and/or psychological treatment (focusing on posttraumatic stress). Contrary to the hypothesis, the multiprofessional early intervention did not result in any significant improvements as compared with usual care. In fact, at the 6-month follow-up, the multiprofessional group had a *higher rate* of nonrecovery than the control! However, the intervention may have resulted in more "medically" oriented treatment as 94% received medications and all received one or more forms of physical therapy. By comparison, only about half actually received the psychological treatment. Taken together, this study shows no significant benefit in providing early medical treatment. Although it is difficult to draw any conclusion, perhaps the additional attention from physicians and physical therapists early on actually reinforced illness beliefs and avoidance behaviors.

Finally, specifically targeting fear avoidance for those who demonstrate these beliefs and behaviors may be a way forward to improve recovery rates after an acute WAD. In general, activation programs are often associated with improved outcome for acute WAD [51]. One would expect that identifying specific fears and treating them within the first weeks after injury might be particularly effective for those with high levels of fear and avoidance.

Chronic Pain-Oriented Rehabilitation

Despite modern medical treatments, half of those who sustain WAD will still experience neck pain 1 year after injury [8]. This is about the same rate as for back pain, where approximately 50% still have pain problems after 12 months and 5–12% develop persistent problems [9, 21, 27]. Indeed, both neck and low back pain top the list of the most burdensome illnesses in the world [61]. Consequently, WAD in many ways resembles the problems reported by people with other forms of musculoskeletal pain, and thus the large literature on neck and back pain has been brought to bear on it. Therefore, patients with WAD have been included in multimodal pain rehabilitation programs, where content varies greatly but is often focused on the pain experience as well as physical and psychological function. It should be mentioned that some programs for those with chronic WAD focus on specific factors (e.g., PTSD or fear avoidance), and these were described in the sections above.

Reviews of the evidence for the rehabilitation of chronic WAD patients recommend a combination of exercises and cognitive-behavioral interventions [39, 43]. However, the results of these efforts have been mixed, and the overall effect appears to be relatively small. For example, 2 studies have examined whether adding CBT to physical therapy is helpful when performed by physical therapists [38, 45]. Both show that physical therapy and physical therapy with the addition of CBT are helpful, but there are few differences between the groups. While there is some speculation that this may be due to the administration and dosage of the CBT [19], it may simply reflect the overall state of treating chronic pain problems. In fact, a recent review of all types of treatments for chronic, noncancer pain shows very modest improvements in pain and minimal improvements in physical and emotional functioning [55, 63]. As a result, there is a need for further research and development and good reason to consider matching treatments to patient needs.

IMPROVING RESULTS: NEW APPLICATIONS

Given the difficulties in successfully treating persistent pain and, in particular, chronic WAD, some new methods have been investigated. In this section, I will describe efforts aimed at matching, and then turn to new interventions aimed at the comorbidity often present when the pain becomes persistent. These are Acceptance and Commitment Therapy (ACT) for pain and hybrid treatment aimed at mutually maintaining factors.

Matching Treatment to Patient Needs

Matching is a simple and enticing idea that tailoring a treatment to the specific needs of the individual patient should produce better results than general programs [4, 33, 54]. Indeed, while a review of the literature found solid evidence for numerous psychological risk factors as well as for several treatment techniques, treatments did not match risk factors [44]. So although matching is an appealing proposal, it is not well researched. This may be because even general treatment programs tend to tailor the program to the needs of the patient. In addition, it has been difficult to isolate key variables to guide the matching process and new assessment instruments that assist in this process worthy of attention [40].

At present, the data on matching for pain problems are not particularly impressive. First, there are few prospective studies in the literature that are actually designed to ascertain the effects of matching. Second, the results are at best mixed and at worst show little effects as compared with other treatment options [17, 18]. Our team recently designed a study where matching three current psychological treatments to patient profiles was compared with randomly assigning patients to one of the three [5]. The results showed no sign of any advantage of the matching, but we could demonstrate that how and when the assessment of key variables is conducted is crucial [4]. Although matching is a prominent tactic, more research is needed to provide an evidence base for routines in how this might best be done.

Targeting Pain and Emotion

Pain and strong emotions often occur together, and both may be driven by transdiagnostic processes like catastrophizing or avoidance [28]. For some patients, the emotional distress the chronic pain produces may be as disruptive as the pain itself. Indeed, the pain and disability may be explained in terms of the avoidance of unpleasant experiences like the pain itself or negative emotions [15, 28, 37]. Therefore, new treatments have focused on providing interventions that focus on different targets than a traditional pain program would have. Here, I focus on 2 studies that represent this approach.

In a first attempt to ascertain whether ACT was of value, patients suffering chronic WAD were randomly assigned to either an ACT intervention or a waiting-list control. Rather than focusing on controlling or avoiding the pain and negative affect, the ACT treatment of 10 sessions focused on shifting perspective and acceptance. At the same time, exposure techniques were utilized to help achieve valued goals. Results showed large and significant improvements for disability, life satisfaction, fear, and depression, but not for pain intensity. Although we do not know whether ACT contributed anything beyond the effects of exposure, this study suggests that the approach needs further investigation before becoming a standard.

Because patients with chronic WAD may also experience emotional disorders, a hybrid treatment that offers treatment to address both problems may be necessary [28]. Our team devised a so-called hybrid treatment that is based partly on exposure and partly on emotion regulation skills training [31]. We noted that many patients undergoing exposure in vivo treatment (see above) did not respond mainly because they were overpowered by negative affect [12, 13]. Therefore, we wanted to provide a package for these patients. Treatment of about 12 hours first focused on reducing negative affect and developing important, personally relevant goals. Then, patients utilized various emotion regulation skills to assist in being able to fulfill exposure treatment. Third, exposure to both avoided movements but also to avoided situations and emotions was conducted, and, finally, a maintenance program was initiated. A controlled single-subject design was employed that showed that all 6 patients improved considerably even though they had previously undergone many unsuccessful treatments. Moreover, 5 of the 6 participants reached reduced levels of catastrophizing, fear, and pain, and improved physical function. While much more evidence is required, the study demonstrates the need to pursue this line of research.

Other Strategies

Although psychological variables have long been implicated in WAD, the development of psychologically informed treatments is still in its infancy. We have seen above that some studies show that psychological methods can be quite helpful. However, some studies show smaller effects, and in no study do all of the patients improve sufficiently. Consequently, there is a need to improve the consistency, size, and maintenance of treatment results.

Improving the results of psychological interventions for WAD might be done in several ways in future research. First, some of the variance in the results appears to be related to inconsistencies in the application of the interventions. Improvements might be achieved by finding out how much treatment is needed, at what time point in the development of the problem, and for what target variable (e.g., fear, physical function, depression, PTSD). Along the same line, more knowledge is needed about the effects of competency in administering psychological treatments.

A second research line might focus on better assessment methods from the first visit to identify psychological factors that might be viable targets in treatment. In our research clinic, for example, we have shown that the early identification of patients with musculoskeletal pain problems is possible and that treating these patients with a cognitive-behavioral intervention prevents the development of disability [29, 30, 35]. Somewhat similar results have also been shown in a program in primary care that stratifies risk levels and provides treatment proportionally [20]. Once methods for screening are implemented, the more treatments as well as matching may be developed further and evaluated. At this point, the matching process appears to be often done in an unsystematic way that more reflects the idiosyncrasies of the clinician than guidance from models or evidence.

A third area in need of more research is the development of specific psychological interventions for psychological targets. I believe that systems could be developed and tested that would utilize basic psychological treatments like emotion regulation skills, exposure techniques, and interventions for PTSD. There seems to be a real need to research which and what combination of these interventions might best be applied to patients diagnosed with WAD in order to maximize outcomes.

A fourth area is research concerning co-occurring problems, since WAD is often associated with other problems (e.g., depression, PTSD, fear, insomnia). Yet there are few programs that actually address multiple problems. As a result, research should test how these co-occurring problems are best dealt with. New methods like ACT and hybrid protocols are in need of further development and evaluation.

A fifth area is improving long-term results (e.g., by adding specific techniques or follow-up programs). Another approach is to incorporate

Phase	Guiding Principle	Clinical Application
Assessment	1. Psychological factors like fear, PTSD symptoms, and depression increase the likelihood of developing a persistent problem, and once chronic, maintain the problem. 2. WAD naturally leads to emotional and behavioral consequences for most patients. 3. Personal goals are important determinants of engagement and outcome.	1. Psychological factors should be included in routine assessment. In proximity to the injury, screening instruments are helpful [23, 34]. Additional assessment may focus on specific psychological factors like fear avoidance, depression, or PTSD. 2. Psychological concepts may be used in psychoeducation and consultation to provide empathy without reinforcing pain behavior. 3. Ascertain the patient's goals, and utilize these in treatment planning.
Treatment planning	1. Different patients may have quite different factors that are driving their problem. 2. Specific psychological factors will emerge for certain patients. 3. Patients hold different beliefs and expectations about treatment.	1. Matching, that is, tailoring the treatment content to the patient, is helpful. 2. When specific factors are pertinent, plan to use standardized psychological methods for the problem. 3. Provide realistic expectations and take beliefs into account.
Treatment implementation	1. To achieve results, patients need to understand and accept the idea of "self-management." 2. Apply known psychological methods for specific problems. 3. If there are co-occurring problems, consider using multiple methods.	1. Focusing too much on diagnostic and biomedical details may reinforce cure seeking. Use psychoeducation to explain the approach, and work with goals to make it relevant. 2. Judicious use of the techniques (qualified delivery, sufficient amount, etc.) provides maximum effect. 3. Use more than one psychological method when indicated (e.g., for function and sleep or depression and pain).

skills training (e.g., in solving problems and renewing goals) in order to achieve long-term progress. However, all of these ideas have yet to be investigated for patients diagnosed with WAD.

CLINICAL RECOMMENDATIONS

Although the evidence is far from complete, I offer some basic clinical recommendations based on the state of the art. Table 12-2 shows these recommendations according to the phase for the intervention, the guiding principles, and the general application in the clinic. These may be applied in a variety of clinical settings and within the framework of a variety of treatment approaches.

CONCLUSION

Psychological approaches to treating WAD include a rich variety of treatments. The evidence suggests that psychological treatments aimed at specific aspects of WAD (e.g., PTSD symptoms, fear of movement, and function) are helpful when professionally applied. The effect sizes recorded for multimodal programs for chronic WAD are quite small. However, several new approaches are being researched (e.g., matching and emotion-focused treatments) that give hope for improvements. When WAD is accompanied by strong psychological and emotional reactions, psychological treatments should be considered that target these problem areas.

REFERENCES

1. Adams H, Ellis T, Stanish WD, Sullivan MJ. Psychosocial factors related to return to work following rehabilitation of whiplash injuries. J Occup Rehabil 2007;17(2):305–15.

2. Bailey KM, Carleton RN, Vlaeyen JW, Asmundson GJ. Treatments addressing pain-related fear and anxiety in patients with chronic musculoskeletal pain: a preliminary review. Cogn Behav Ther 2010;39(1):46–63.

3. Barrera T, Mott J, Hofstein R, Teng E. A meta-analytic review of exposure in group cognitive behavioral therapy for posttraumatic stress disorder. Clin Psychol Rev 2013;33(1):24–32.

4. Bergbom S, Boersma K, Linton SJ. When matching fails: understanding the process of matching pain-disability treatment to risk profile. J Occup Rehabil 2014; Epub Dec 11.

5. Bergbom S, Flink IK, Boersma K, Linton SJ. Early psychologically informed interventions for workers at risk for pain-related disability: does matching treatment to profile improve outcome? J Occup Rehabil 2014;24:446–57.

6. Bisson J, Andrew M. Psychological treatment of post-traumatic stress disorder (PTSD). Cochrane Database Syst Rev 2007;(3):CD003388.

7. Blanchard EB, Hickling EJ, Freidenberg BM, Malta LS, Kuhn E, Sykes MA. Two studies of psychiatric morbidity among motor vehicle accident survivors 1 year after the crash. Behav Res Ther 2004;42(5):569–83.

8. Carroll LJ, Holm LW, Hogg-Johnson S, Côtè P, Cassidy JD, Haldeman S, Nordin M, Hurwitz EL, Carragee EJ, van der Velde G, et al. Course and prognostic factors for neck pain in whiplash-associated disorders (WAD): results of the Bone and Joint Decade 2000–2010 Task Force on Neck Pain and Its Associated Disorders. J Manipulative Physiol Ther 2009;32(2, Suppl):S97–S107.

9. Crombie IK, Croft PR, Linton SJ, LeResche L, Von Korff M. Epidemiology of pain. Seattle, WA: International Association for the Study of Pain Press; 1999.

10. de Jong JR, Vangronsveld K, Peters ML, Goossens ME, Onghena P, Bulté I, Vlaeyen JW. Reduction of pain-related fear and disability in post-traumatic neck pain: a replicated single-case experimental study of exposure in vivo. J Pain 2008;9(12):1123–34.

11. Dunne RL, Kenardy J, Sterling M. A randomized controlled trial of cognitive-behavioral therapy for the treatment of PTSD in the context of chronic whiplash. Clin J Pain 2012;28(9):755–65.

12. Flink I, Boersma K, Linton S. When treatment fails; exposure is less helpful for pain catastrophizers. Eur J Pain 2009;13(Suppl 1):S265c–S266.

13. Flink I, Boersma K, Linton S. Catastrophizing moderates the effect of exposure in vivo for back pain patients with pain-related fear. Eur J Pain 2010;14(8):887–92.

14. Flink I, Boersma K, Linton SJ. Pain catastrophizing as repetitive negative thinking: a development of the conceptualization. Cogn Behav Ther 2013;42(3):215–23.

15. Fordyce WE. Behavioral methods for chronic pain and illness. St. Louis, MO: Mosby; 1976.

16. Freedman SA, Shalev AY. Is prevention better than cure? How early interventions can prevent PTSD. In: Safir MP, Wallach HS, Rizzo A, editors. Future directions in post-traumatic stress disorder. New York, NY: Springer; 2015. pp. 171–86.

17. Gatchel RJ, Noe CE, Pulliam C, Robbins H, Deschner M, Gajraj NM, Vakharia AS. A preliminary study of multidimensional pain inventory profile differences in predicting treatment outcome in a heterogeneous cohort of patients with chronic pain. Clin J Pain 2002;18(3):139–43.

18. George SZ, Fritz JM, Bialosky JE, Donald DA. The effect of a fear-avoidance–based physical therapy intervention for patients with acute low back pain: results of a randomized clinical trial. Spine 2003;28(23):2551–60.

19. Gross AR, Kaplan F, Huang S, Khan M, Santaguida PL, Carlesso LC, Macdermid JC, Walton DM, Kenardy J, Söderlund A, et al. Psychological care, patient education, orthotics, ergonomics and prevention strategies for neck pain: an systematic overview update as part of the ICON Project. Open Orthop J 2013;7:530–61.

20. Hill JC, Whitehurst DG, Lewis M, Bryan S, Dunn KM, Foster NE, Konstantinou K, Main CJ, Mason E, Somerville S, et al. Comparison of stratified primary care management for low back pain with current best practice (STarT Back): a randomised controlled trial. Lancet 2011;378:1560–71.

21. Hoy DG, Bain C, Williams G, March L, Brooks P, Blyth F, Woolf A, Vos T, Buchbinder R. A systematic review of the global prevalence of low back pain. Arthritis Rheum 2012;64:2028–37.

22. Jull G, Kenardy J, Hendrikz J, Cohen M, Sterling M. Management of acute whiplash: a randomized controlled trial of multidisciplinary stratified treatments. Pain 2013;154(9):1798–806.

23. Kasch H, Kongsted A, Qerama E, Bach FW, Bendix T, Jensen TS. A new stratified risk assessment tool for whiplash injuries developed from a prospective observational study. BMJ Open 2013;3(1):e002050.

24. Kearns MC, Ressler KJ, Zatzick D, Rothbaum BO. Early interventions for PTSD: a review. Depress Anxiety 2012;29(10):833–42.

25. Linton SJ. New avenues for the prevention of chronic musculoskeletal pain and disability, Vol. 1. Amsterdam: Elsevier; Science 2002.

26. Linton SJ. Why does chronic pain develop? A behavioral approach. In: Linton SJ, editor. New avenues for the prevention of chronic musculoskeletal pain and disability. Amsterdam: Elsevier; 2002. pp. 67–82.

27. Linton SJ. Understanding pain for better clinical practice. Edinburgh: Elsevier; 2005.

28. Linton SJ. A transdiagnostic approach to pain and emotion. J Appl Biobehav Res 2013;18(2):82–103.

29. Linton SJ, Andersson T. Can chronic disability be prevented? A randomized trial of a cognitive-behavior intervention and two forms of information for patients with spinal pain. Spine 2000;25(21):2825–31.

30. Linton SJ, Boersma K, Traczyk M, Shaw WS, Nicholas M. Early workplace communication and problem solving to prevent back disability: results of a randomized controlled trial among high-risk workers and their supervisors. J Occup Rehabil 2015; Epub Jul 23.

31. Linton SJ, Fruzzetti A. A hybrid emotion-focused exposure treatment for chronic pain: a feasibility study. Scand J Pain 2014;5(3):151–8.

32. Linton SJ, Gross D, Schultz IZ, Main CJ, Côté P, Pransky G, Johnson W. Prognosis and the identification of workers risking disability. J Occup Rehabil 2005;15(4):459–74.

33. Linton SJ, Nicholas MK. After assessment then what? Integrating findings for successful case formulation and treatment tailoring. In: Breivik H, Campbell WI, Nicholas MK, editors. Clinical pain management: practice and procedures. London: Hodder & Stoughton; 2008. pp. 95–106.

34. Linton SJ, Nicholas M, MacDonald S. Development of a short form of the Örebro Musculoskeletal Pain Screening Questionnaire. Spine 2011;36(22):1891–5.

35. Linton SJ, Nordin E. A 5-year follow-up evaluation of the health and economic consequences of an early cognitive behavioral intervention for back pain: a randomized, controlled trial. Spine 2006;31(8):853–8.

36. Lohnberg JA. A review of outcome studies on cognitive-behavioral therapy for reducing fear-avoidance beliefs among Individuals with chronic pain. J Clin Psychol Med Settings 2007;14:113–22.

37. McCracken LM, Morley S. The psychological flexibility model: a basis for integration and progress in psychological approaches to chronic pain management. J Pain 2014;15(3):221–34.

38. Monticone M, Baiardi P, Vanti C, Ferrari S, Nava T, Montironi C, Rocca B, Foti C, Teli M. Chronic neck pain and treatment of cognitive and behavioural factors: results of a randomised controlled clinical trial. Eur Spine J 2012;21(8):1558–66.

39. Nijs J, Van Oosterwijck J, De Hertogh W. Rehabilitation of chronic whiplash: treatment of cervical dysfunctions or chronic pain syndrome? Clin Rheumatol 2009;28(3):243–51.

40. Reme SE, Shaw WS, Steenstra IA, Woiszwillo MJ, Pransky G, Linton SJ. Distressed, immobilized, or lacking employer support? A sub-classification of acute work-related low back pain. J Occup Rehabil 2012;22:1–12.

41. Robinson JP, Theodore BR, Dansie EJ, Wilson HD, Turk DC. The role of fear of movement in subacute whiplash-associated disorders grades I and II. Pain 2013;154(3):393–401.

42. Rose SC, Bisson J, Churchill R, Wessely S. Psychological debriefing for preventing post traumatic stress disorder (PTSD). Cochrane Database Syst Rev 2002;(2):CD000560.

43. Seferiadis A, Rosenfeld M, Gunnarsson R. A review of treatment interventions in whiplash-associated disorders. Eur Spine J 2004;13(5):387–97.

44. Shaw WS, Linton SJ, Pransky G. Reducing sickness absence from work due to low back pain: how well do intervention strategies match modifiable risk factors? J Occup Rehabil 2006;16:591–605.

45. Soderlund A, Lindberg P. Cognitive behavioural components in physiotherapy management of chronic whiplash associated disorders (WAD)—a randomised group study. G Ital Med Lav Ergon 2007;29(1, Suppl A):A5–A11.

46. Spitzer WO, Skovron ML, Salmi LR, Cassidy JD, Suissa S, Zeiss E. Scientific monograph of the Quebec Task Force on whiplash-associated disorders: redefining "whiplash" and its management. Spine 1995;20:S1–S70.

47. Sterling M. Physiotherapy management of whiplash-associated disorders (WAD). J Physiother 2014;60(1):5–12.

48. Sullivan M, Adams H, Horan S, Maher D, Boland D, Gross R. The role of perceived injustice in the experience of chronic pain and disability: scale development and validation. J Occup Rehabil 2008;18(3):249–61.

49. Sullivan M, Adams H, Rhodenizer T, Stanish W. A psychosocial risk factor—targeted intervention for the prevention of chronic pain and disability following whiplash injury. Phys Ther 2006;86(1):8–18.

50. Sullivan MJ, Thibault P, Simmonds MJ, Milioto M, Cantin A-P, Velly AM. Pain, perceived injustice and the persistence of post-traumatic stress symptoms during the course of rehabilitation for whiplash injuries. Pain 2009;145(3):325–31.

51. Teasell RW, McClure JA, Walton D, Pretty J, Salter K, Meyer M, Sequeira K, Death B. A research synthesis of therapeutic interventions for whiplash-associated disorder (WAD), Part 2: interventions for acute WAD. Pain Res Manag 2010;15(5):295–304.

52. Trost Z, Vangronsveld K, Linton SJ, Quartana PJ, Sullivan MJ. Cognitive dimensions of anger in chronic pain. Pain 2012;153(3):515–7.

53. Turk DC. Chronic pain and whiplash associated disorders: rehabilitation and secondary prevention. Pain Res Manag 2003;8:40–3.

54. Turk DC. The potential of treatment matching for subgroups of patients with chronic pain: lumping versus splitting. Clin J Pain 2005;21(1):44–55.

55. Turk DC, Wilson HD, Cahana A. Treatment of chronic non-cancer pain. Lancet 2011;377(9784):2226–35.

56. Van Damme S, Legrain V, Vogt J, Crombez G. Keeping pain in mind: a motivational account of attention to pain. Neurosci Biobehav Rev 2010;34(2):204–13.

57. Vernon H, Mior S. The Neck Disability Index: a study of reliability and validity. J Manipulative Physiol Ther 1991;14(7):409–15.

58. Vlaeyen JW, Linton SJ. Fear-avoidance and its consequences in chronic musculoskeletal pain: a state of the art. Pain 2000;85:317–32.

59. Vlaeyen JW, Linton SJ. Fear-avoidance model of chronic musculoskeletal pain: 12 years on. Pain 2012;153:1144–7.

60. Vlaeyen JW, Morely SJ, Linton SJ, Boersma K, de Jong J. Pain-related fear: exposure-based treatment for chronic pain. Seattle, WA: International Association for the Study of Pain; 2012.

61. Vos T, Flaxman AD, Naghavi M, Lozano R, Michaud C, Ezzati M, Shibuya K, Salomon JA, Abdalla S, Aboyans V, et al. Years lived with disability (YLDs) for 1160 sequelae of 289 diseases and injuries 1990–2010: a systematic analysis for the Global Burden of Disease Study 2010. Lancet 2013;380(9859):2163–96.

62. Wicksell RK, Ahlqvist J, Bring A, Melin L, Olsson GL. Can exposure and acceptance strategies improve functioning and life satisfaction in people with chronic pain and whiplash-associated disorders (WAD)? A randomized controlled trial. Cogn Behav Ther 2008;37(3):169–82.

63. Williams A, Eccleston C, Morley S. Psychological therapies for the management of chronic pain (excluding headache) in adults. Cochrane Database Syst Rev 2012; (2):CD007407.

CHAPTER 13

Precollision Risk Factors, Illness-Related Cognition, and Recovery After Acute Whiplash Trauma

Tina Birgitte Wisbech Carstensen and Lisbeth Frostholm

Persistent pain and disability after whiplash trauma has become an increasingly significant problem in many industrialized countries as it has comprehensive individual as well as social costs in terms of the patients' impaired physiological, psychological, economic, and domestic conditions [3, 22]. Of course, those consequences are prevalent in most chronic illnesses. The curious thing about WAD is that the above-mentioned pervasive consequences arise from a relatively minor impact. No dose–response relationship between trauma intensity and subsequent disablement has been shown, and several studies now point to collision severity being of minor importance [3, 6, 17]. Theoretically, cervical sprain (acute whiplash trauma) heals approximately within the same time frame as an ankle sprain, but a substantial proportion of the whiplash-exposed continue to experience symptoms [20].

This gives rise to an interesting question: Why is the impact substantial for some individuals, leaving them with persistent symptoms and disability, whereas for others, it is merely an experience of transient pain? Most acute whiplash-exposed do recover within the first

3 months, and after this time, the recovery rates level off [19]. Despite an exponential increase in research on whiplash during the last sixty years, we still miss substantial pieces of the puzzle.

A BIOPSYCHOSOCIAL PERSPECTIVE ON WHIPLASH

There is strong evidence to suggest that people's self-rated health and psychosocial factors influence morbidity and mortality independent of biomedical disease parameters [9]. In whiplash research, a biopsychosocial model was introduced in the 1990s by Ferrari and Russell [11][1]. Up till then, consequences of the whiplash trauma on the neck (muscles, skeleton, ligaments, etc.) had primarily been seen as the cause of persistent symptoms. The biopsychosocial approach presents several physiological factors (acute neck sprain, inexpedient posture as a reaction to pain, etc.) as the basis for the development of symptoms after whiplash trauma. Ferrari et al. [10], stressed that physiological factors may be viewed as the base on which the psychological factors operate, and physiological factors may elicit the psychological factors, for example, perception of symptoms and reactions to pain (coping strategies), and these reactions can be maladaptive or adaptive. However, there is an ever growing awareness that biopsychosocial interrelationships are much more complicated.

PREDISPOSING, TRIGGERING, AND PERPETUATING FACTORS

Broadly speaking, the factors involved in developing chronic WAD can be classified into predisposing, triggering, or perpetuating factors

---

[1] "Bio" in the word "biopsychosocial" may refer to the words somatic/physiological /biological/ bodily. However, when experiencing a so-called "physiological symptom" following an injury, we know that there is already substantial psychology involved in that experience. The International Association for the Study of Pain (IASP) defines pain as follows: An unpleasant sensory and emotional experience associated with actual or potential tissue damage, or described in terms of such damage. Hence, the words physiological and psychological factors should not be used as these words imply an implicit dualism. However, this is the prevalent terminology as no other fulfilling alternative has yet been proposed.

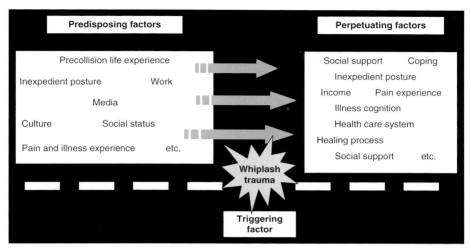

FIGURE 13-1 Multifactorial model of whiplash trauma.

(Fig. 13-1). According to this model, the individual enters the motor vehicle collision as a person from a certain culture, having accumulated experience with health and illness that might leave the individual at risk for developing persistent pain. The whiplash trauma may trigger certain vulnerability factors and interact together with social, psychological, and physiological perpetuating factors after the accident in the course of developing persistent pain after whiplash trauma.

PRECOLLISION RISK FACTORS

Most research within whiplash has focused on collision-related factors and factors after the collision. Recently, researchers have started to look into factors before the accident to explore predisposing factors that influence recovery. It has been suggested that physiological and psychological vulnerability before the accident may to some extent explain the varied response to acute whiplash trauma [21, 22].

Precollision Social Risk Factors

Only a few studies have explored precollision social factors as risk factors for poor recovery following whiplash trauma. In 2008, a meta-analysis and a best evidence synthesis concluded that no scientifically admissible studies exploring the effect of social factors on the onset of persistent symptoms following whiplash trauma existed [17, 19]. One of the few social factors that have been studied is the impact of education on recovery. However, these findings are heterogeneous. Some reviews conclude that low education is associated with negative outcome [26], and other reviews present no association or diverging results on associations with recovery [3, 8]. The impact of other precollision socioeconomic factors has been explored. Some studies suggest that unemployment [6] and low family income [16] increase the risk of poor recovery, while other studies find no association between poor recovery and prior earnings [22].

Only two studies have explored the impact of receiving welfare benefits before the whiplash trauma, for example, sick pay and disability pension. Myrtveit et al. [24] retrieved self-reported data on welfare benefits and the latter from a national register on welfare benefits. They found that short-term health-related benefits increased the risk of chronic neck pain by 65%, while long-term health-related benefits and unemployment benefits did not predict recovery [24]. We found that receiving accumulated sickness benefit of 12 weeks or more during a five-year period before the accident was associated with both negative change in provisional situation OR (CI) = 3.8 (2.1;7.1) and considerable neck pain OR (CI) = 3.3 (1.8;6.3) 1 year after the accident [5]. Receiving unemployment benefit and social assistance within the last 5 years before the accident did not predict future negative change in provisional situation or neck pain [5]. These findings suggest that receiving short-term health-related benefits as sick pay before the collision is an important risk factor for poor recovery following whiplash trauma regardless of data being self-rated or obtained from other sources.

Precollision Psychological Risk Factors

A range of studies have examined the association between precollision psychological distress (e.g., previous psychological problems, anxiety, depression, psychiatric factors) and recovery [8, 21], and reviews state that results are inconclusive [27]. The focus, however, has been on single specific psychological dimensions or disorders (e.g., anxiety or depression), and only a few studies have explored accumulated precollision psychological distress. We found that experiencing accumulated psychological distress before the collision predicted poor recovery 1 year after the collision OR (CI) = 2.1 (1.1;4.2) [6]. Surprisingly, poor recovery was predicted solely if distress was accumulated of several psychological distress factors. Most of the individuals experiencing accumulated distress showed symptoms of more than five out of seven psychological problems (anxiety, depression, hostility, obsessive compulsive disorder, somatization, emotional psychiatric disorder, illness worry). 11.4% ($n = 84$) of this cohort of persons with acute whiplash had precollision accumulated psychological distress. However, accumulated psychological distress was only found to predict future neck pain and did not affect work capability 1 year after the accident. Psychological distress before the collision might be a predisposing factor for poor recovery, in particular accumulation of psychological distress, but these findings have to be replicated and explored in other cohorts of patients with whiplash.

Precollision Physiological Risk Factors

With respect to precollision physiological factors, research has indicated that some of the strongest associations with poor recovery are factors that are present before the accident, for example, back pain [21], neck pain [1, 6, 26], unspecified pain [1, 6], self-rated poor general health [1, 16, 24], high frequency of attendance to general practitioner [1, 21], high use of health care [22, 24], and use of medications [24]. High levels of physical fitness before the collision have been shown to be a protecting factor [14, 24]. It can be disputed whether, for example, pain and use of medical care can be seen as physiological factors, as there is substantial psychology involved in these issues.

A meta-analysis showed a small but statistically significant negative effect of precollision neck pain on recovery [26]. Research has tended to focus on specific pain (e.g., neck pain, headache) rather than widespread or unspecified pain. To our knowledge, only two studies have explored the prognostic value of precollision unspecified pain. Atherton et al. [1] found that whiplash patients with widespread pain during the previous month before the collision had a higher risk (RR: 1.8) of persistent neck pain 1 year after the collision. Similarly, we found that reporting a pain condition entailing sick report 2 weeks or more during the 5 years before the collision was a risk factor of great significance [6]. 23.5% ($n = 169$) of this cohort of persons with acute whiplash had a precollision pain condition. Pain condition predicted (1) future neck pain, (2) reduced work capability, and (3) negative change in provisional situation [5, 6].

Persistent pain after whiplash trauma falls within the cluster of pain conditions that are termed idiopathic, that is, the cause of pain is unknown. There is no demonstrable tissue injury or inflammation. These are also called functional pain conditions. A central sensitization in the nervous system has been proposed to partly explain persistent pain following whiplash trauma, and sensitization in pain conditions such as chronic WAD has been reported [20, 25].

THE TRANSITION FROM ACUTE TO CHRONIC PAIN

As we can see, emerging evidence supports the view that certain precollision factors have an impact on the development of chronic WAD. Theoretically, however, if we do not wish merely to understand those precollision factors as the basis on which the whiplash trauma and the perpetuating factors operate, we lack a better account of how predisposing, triggering, and perpetuating factors may dynamically interact. We propose that the CSM may provide exactly such a framework.

THE COMMON-SENSE MODEL (CSM) OF ILLNESS

According to the CSM, people act as "common-sense scientists" when they use concrete experience of symptoms to create an understanding of a health threat. The processing of a health threat takes place in sequential but recursive stages from the initial perception of symptoms

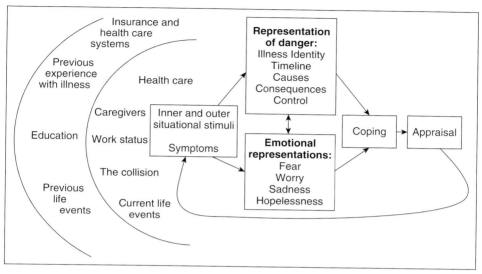

FIGURE 13-2 The common-sense model of illness.

through coping to appraisal of the actions taken to solve the health problem (Fig. 13-2).

When a person is exposed to acute whiplash trauma, he or she develops a set of organized beliefs, also called illness perceptions, about the trauma. These beliefs are shaped in a dynamic process in which both actual experiences with the symptoms, caregivers, health care, and so on as well as previous experiences with health and illness, and social and cultural assumptions about the trauma play a role.

ILLNESS PERCEPTION COMPONENTS

The CSM provides a more detailed description of the components that have generally been found in peoples' illness models. People organize their understanding around generic components such as illness identity (symptoms and illness label), cause, timeline, perceived control, and expected consequences. Even though the generality of components has been discussed, they have proved fairly consistent both over time and in various illnesses [15].

ILLNESS PERCEPTION IN WAD

In the following, we will provide a brief introduction to the five main components of the CSM, and identify studies that have directly or indirectly examined those components in WAD. We will not specifically target coping strategies, but include them only if they may be considered as belonging within the framework of the following five components.

In a large prospective cohort study of 740 patients exposed to acute whiplash trauma, we included a revised Danish version of the Illness Perception Questionnaire [13]. We obtained patients' perceptions of the symptoms they experienced in the days following the collision, and 3 and 12 months later (Table 13-1).

Overall, we found significant differences at baseline between the illness perceptions of those who continued to develop chronic WAD and those who did not. At baseline, the illness perceptions of both groups are quite comparable to the perceptions of primary care patients consulting with physical health problems [12], with the exception of the illness identity and emotional representations component of the later WAD patients, which are somewhat higher. However, the 1-year follow-up scores of the WAD patients are comparable to or even higher than those of primary care patients with a diagnosed somatoform disorder (ibid).

Illness identity refers to the label (e.g., a whiplash trauma) and the associated symptoms (e.g., neck pain, headache). Buitenhuis et al. [2] found that persons labeling neck symptoms after motor vehicle accidents as "whiplash" were more likely to report disability 1 year after the collision. The label is the backbone of the other illness components, and the importance of a label is elucidated by the frustrations experienced by patients faced with diagnostic uncertainty. In WAD, there is much confusion and uncertainty regarding how to understand the illness, which may incline the patient to rely on lay sources to make sense of the symptoms.

Overall, the transition from acute to chronic whiplash may be regarded as a process in which the illness identity of the patient gets increasingly stronger with more and more general symptoms being associated with whiplash. We found that patients who developed chronic pain experienced significantly more symptoms in the week after the

TABLE 13-1 Illness Perceptions by Neck Pain 1 Year After Acute Whiplash Trauma*

	Self-reported Neck Pain on a 11 Point Box Scale 1 Year After the Collision		
	Neck Pain <4 (0–10) N = 340	Neck Pain ≥4 (0–10) N = 189	Test of Equality of Means
SOCIODEMOGRAPHICS			
Gender (% females)	61.5	77.3	$X^2(1) = 13.7, P < 0.0001$
Age (18–65), mean (SD)	35.8 (11.8)	36.1 (11.6)	$Z = 0.26, P = 0.611$
Education (%)			
White collar and employed	51.5	41.8	
Blue collar	18.8	25.4	
Student	19.7	19.6	
Unemployed	7.7	11.1	
Unaccounted	2.4	2.1	$X^2(4) = 6.5, P = 0.164$
ILLNESS PERCEPTIONS*	**Mean (SD)**	**Mean (SD)**	**Kruskal Wallis**
Illness identity (0–12 symptoms)[†]			
Baseline n = 339/189[‡]	**2.6** (2.1)	**3.4** (2.4)	$Z = 13.2, P = 0.003$
3 months n = 305/168	**3.8** (2.6)	**6.8** (2.7)	$Z = 98.1, P < 0.001$
12 months n = 328/184	**3.4** (2.6)	**6.6** (2.9)	$Z = 119.6, P < 0.001$
Consequences (0–100)			
Baseline n = 329/186	**6.6** (12.3)	**12.3** (19.1)	$Z = 8.4, P = 0.004$
3 months n = 288/160	**8.3** (15.5)	**30.7** (28.7)	$Z = 80.4, P < 0.001$
12 months n = 314/171	**6.6** (16.4)	**39.2** (31.4)	$Z = 139.9, P < 0.001$
Emotional representations (0–100)			
Baseline n = 329/186	**15.8** (17.9)	**27.1** (25.2)	$Z = 24.8, P < 0.001$
3 months n = 288/160	**9.2** (15.4)	**30.5** (28.0)	$Z = 71.3, P < 0.001$
12 months n = 314/171	**5.0** (12.6)	**33.3** (30.5)	$Z = 136.2, P < 0.001$
Long timeline perspective (0–100)			
Baseline n = 329/186	**13.9** (17.2)	**20.4** (23.9)	$Z = 6.2, P = 0.013$
3 months n = 288/160	**18.5** (23.8)	**38.3** (33.2)	$Z = 39.5, P < 0.001$
12 months n = 314/171	**13.9** (24.7)	**56.3** (32.9)	$Z = 154.7, P < 0.001$
Personal control (0–100)			
Baseline n = 329/186	83.6 (16.9)	84.2 (16.9)	$Z = 0.2, P = 0.691$
3 months n = 288/160	**81.1** (21.0)	**72.5** (22.9)	$Z = 18.4, P < 0.001$
12 months n = 314/171	**77.5** (15.5)	**62.9** (23.6)	$Z = 56.4, P < 0.001$

*Obtained by questionnaire within 2 weeks after the collision, and 3 and 12 months after the collision. For details on components and scoring of components see Frostholm et al. [12].
[†]The SCL-12—a 12-item check list on physical symptoms used as a proxy measure of illness identity.
[‡]Number of participants completing the component in the low and high neck pain group.

accident and that this seemed to be settled 3 months after the collision with a large difference in experienced symptoms between the two groups (Table 13-1).

Timeline perspective refers to beliefs regarding the duration of the symptoms and can be short lasting, cyclical, or chronic. We found that patients who did not expect to return to work within 6 weeks after the collision had an increased risk of having reduced working ability 1 year after the collision [13]. Chronic WAD patients had a significantly stronger belief in a long duration of the symptoms already at baseline, a difference that increased considerably from baseline to 1 year later (Table 13-1).

Consequences refer to the individual's ideas about the impact of illness. The consequence component has generally been shown to be a powerful predictor of health outcomes in various illnesses. This component shares a conceptual overlap with pain catastrophizing, which has been shown to be a very consistent predictor of poor recovery in WAD [5, 26]. Holm et al. [18] found a dose–response relationship between recovery expectations and disability in acute WAD; that is, those with the lowest expectations for recovery had the poorest recovery, and those with the highest expectations had the best recovery. In line with this, we found a stronger belief in negative consequences at all time points for patients with chronic WAD (Table 13-1).

Causal attributions are closely associated with our efforts to make sense of illness. When health care professionals provide a diagnosis, some notion of causality is often offered, but patients often have their own perceptions of causality, which do not match those of the health care system. Buitenhuis et al. [2] found that people reporting neck pain after motor vehicle accidents were more likely to experience disability when they perceived "a severe injury" to be the cause of their symptoms.

Control reflects both the individual's experience of having the power to influence the symptoms (i.e., personal control) and the individual's belief in the beneficial effect of treatment (i.e., treatment control). Using the 3-item measure of personal control from a condensed Danish version of the IPQ, we found differences at 3 and 12 months after the collision between patients with and without WAD (Table 13-1).

However, in a recently published study using a simple 9-item measure on coping and treatment preferences, we found that treatment preferences for medication and sick leave were associated with neck pain and reduced work ability 1 year later [23]. In addition, active coping preferences such as to keep going as normal and changing lifestyle reduced the odds of disability 1 year later (ibid).

Emotional representations concern the emotions that the individual perceives as related to the health threat and have been found to be moderate to highly correlated with the consequences dimension. Previous research has found depressed mood [3] and posttraumatic stress symptoms [27] to predict disability. More specifically, in accordance with the CSM, Carroll et al. [4] found that each pain-related emotion increased the risk of developing chronic WAD. We found a much larger score on the emotional representations component at baseline for patients who later developed chronic WAD compared with patients who did not (Table 13-1).

An illness perception index: To examine whether illness perceptions predicted chronic WAD, we estimated an index of the three components that have been found to be the strongest predictors of disability in previous studies using the CSM: consequences, long timeline, and emotional representations [13]. Patients obtaining a high score on this index during the first week after the collision were more likely to develop chronic neck pain, OR (CI) = 3.4 (1.5;7.8). A high score on the same index 3 months after the collision were associated with chronic neck pain at 12 months, OR (CI) = 8.6 (4.4;16.9). To get an estimate of the impact of this index in combination with other examined risk factors, we estimated that a 40-year-old woman with a low educational level, high neck pain at baseline, and a score of 0 on the IP index had a 55%, 95% CI (45%;64%) probability of chronic neck pain, whereas a woman with the same characteristics but with a score of 2 on the IP baseline index had an 81%, 95% CI (64%;91%) probability of chronic neck pain (ibid).

The above findings support the notion that the CSM may be a useful framework for understanding the illness trajectory from acute to chronic neck pain. However, we cannot determine whether those illness perceptions are part of the causal pathway of illness development or whether they are markers of other characteristics that directly affect outcome.

CONCLUSIONS AND PERSPECTIVES

This chapter has presented findings on social, psychological, and physiological predisposing factors before the collision. These findings support a complex interrelationship of a range of predisposing factors that may constitute a vulnerability that can be triggered by the whiplash trauma. We propose that the CSM of illness provides a theoretical framework for future intervention studies. This theoretical framework provides a unifying model to help us understand the interaction of predisposing, triggering, and perpetuating factors in the course of developing persistent pain and disability after whiplash trauma.

Taking the above perspective, there may be an array of factors involved in the individual's attempts to handle a condition for which very diverse understandings exist in Western society. Predisposing factors make strong predictors of recovery, and if maladaptive, they form a potential vulnerability in the individual. We need to look further into these vulnerability factors and their connection to the formation of illness perceptions. There seems to be a window within the first 3 months after the collision, in which the illness perceptions are not yet settled in a negative and chronic illness model. In this time frame, interventions aimed at examining, working with, or changing patients' illness models may help prevent the transition from acute to chronic condition.

FUNDING

The study [6, 7, 13, 23] was supported by the trade organization of Insurance and Pensions in Denmark, The Health Insurance Foundation, The Research Foundation of Aarhus University, The Tryg Foundation, The Illum Foundation, The Lippmann Foundation, The Foundation of The Family Hede Nielsen, and The Danish Rheumatism

Association. The funders had no role in the study design, data collection and analysis, decision to publish, or preparation of the manuscript. No information about results or participation in the project was given to the participants' insurance company.

CONFLICT OF INTEREST

The authors have declared that no conflict of interest exist.

REFERENCES

1. Atherton K, Wiles NJ, Lecky FE, Hawes SJ, Silman AJ, Macfarlane GJ, Jones GT. Predictors of persistent neck pain after whiplash injury. Emerg Med J 2006;23:195–201.

2. Buitenhuis J, de Jong PJ, Jaspers JP, Groothoff JW. Work disability after whiplash: a prospective cohort study. Spine (Phila Pa 1976) 2009;34:262–7.

3. Carroll LJ, Holm LW, Hogg-Johnson S, Côté P, Cassidy JD, Haldeman S, Nordin M, Hurwitz EL, Carragee EJ, van der Velde G, et al. Course and prognostic factors for neck pain in whiplash-associated disorders (WAD): results of the Bone and Joint Decade 2000–2010 Task Force on Neck Pain and Its Associated Disorders. Spine 2008;33:S83–S92.

4. Carroll LJ, Liu Y, Holm LW, Cassidy JD, Cote P. Pain-related emotions in early stages of recovery in whiplash-associated disorders: their presence, intensity, and association with pain recovery. Psychosom Med 2011;73:708–15.

5. Carstensen TB, Fink P, Oernboel E, Kasch H, Jensen TS, Frostholm L. Sick leave within 5 years of whiplash trauma predicts recovery: a prospective cohort and register-based study. PLoS One 2015;10(6):e0130298.

6. Carstensen TB, Frostholm L, Oernboel E, Kongsted A, Kasch H, Jensen TS, Fink P. Post-trauma ratings of pre-collision pain and psychological distress predict poor outcome following acute whiplash trauma: a 12-month follow-up study. Pain 2008;139: 248–59.

7. Carstensen TB, Frostholm L, Oernboel E, Kongsted A, Kasch H, Jensen TS, Fink P. Are there gender differences in coping with neck pain following acute whiplash trauma? A 12-month follow-up study. Eur J Pain 2011;16:49–60.

8. Cassidy JD, Carroll LJ, Cote P, Lemstra M, Berglund A, Nygren A. Effect of eliminating compensation for pain and suffering on the outcome of insurance claims for whiplash injury. N Engl J Med 2000;342:1179–86.

9. DeSalvo KB, Bloser N, Reynolds K, He J, Muntner P. Mortality prediction with a single general self-rated health question. A meta-analysis. J Gen Intern Med 2006;21:267–75.

10. Ferrari R, Kwan O, Russell AS, Pearce JM, Schrader H. The best approach to the problem of whiplash? One ticket to Lithuania, please. Clin Exp Rheumatol 1999;17:321–6.

11. Ferrari R, Russell AS. The whiplash syndrome—common sense revisited. J Rheumatol 1997;24:618–23.

12. Frostholm L, Petrie KJ, Ornbol E, Fink P. Are illness perceptions related to future healthcare expenditure in patients with somatoform disorders? Psychol Med 2014;44:2903–11.

13. Gehrt TB, Wisbech Carstensen TB, Ørnbøl E, Fink PK, Kasch H, Frostholm L. The role of illness perceptions in predicting outcome after acute whiplash trauma: a multicenter 12-month follow-up study. Clin J Pain 2015;31:14–20.

14. Geldman M, Moore A, Cheek L. The effect of pre-injury physical fitness on the initial severity and recovery from whiplash injury, at six-month follow-up. Clin Rehabil 2008;22:364–76.

15. Hagger MS, Orbell S. A meta-analytic review of the common-sense model of illness representations. Psychol Health 2003;18:141–84.

16. Holm LW, Carroll LJ, Cassidy JD, Ahlbom A. Factors influencing neck pain intensity in whiplash-associated disorders. Spine (Phila Pa 1976) 2006;31:E98–E104.

17. Holm LW, Carroll LJ, Cassidy JD, Hogg-Johnson S, Côté P, Guzman J, Peloso P, Nordin M, Hurwitz E, van der Velde G, et al. The burden and determinants of neck pain in whiplash-associated disorders after traffic collisions: results of the Bone and Joint Decade 2000–2010 Task Force on Neck Pain and Its Associated Disorders. Spine 2008;33:S52–S59.

18. Holm LW, Carroll LJ, Cassidy JD, Skillgate E, Ahlbom A. Expectations for recovery important in the prognosis of whiplash injuries. PLoS Med 2008;5:e105.

19. Kamper SJ, Rebbeck TJ, Maher CG, McAuley JH, Sterling M. Course and prognostic factors of whiplash: a systematic review and meta-analysis. Pain 2008;138:617–29.

20. Kasch H, Qerama E, Bach FW, Jensen TS. Reduced cold pressor pain tolerance in non-recovered whiplash patients: a 1-year prospective study. Eur J Pain 2005;9:561–9.

21. Lankester BJ, Garneti N, Gargan MF, Bannister GC. Factors predicting outcome after whiplash injury in subjects pursuing litigation. Eur Spine J 2006;15:902–7.

22. Leth-Petersen S, Rotger GP. Long-term labour-market performance of whiplash claimants. J Health Econ 2009;28:996–1011.

23. Myrtveit SM, Carstensen T, Kasch H, Ornbol E, Frostholm L. Initial healthcare and coping preferences are associated with outcome 1 year after whiplash trauma: a multicentre 1-year follow-up study. BMJ Open 2015;5:e007239.

24. Myrtveit SM, Wilhelmsen I, Petrie KJ, Skogen JC, Sivertsen B. What characterizes individuals developing chronic whiplash?: The Nord-Trondelag Health Study (HUNT). J Psychosom Res 2013;74:393–400.

25. Van OJ, Nijs J, Meeus M, Paul L. Evidence for central sensitization in chronic whiplash: a systematic literature review. Eur J Pain 2013;17:299–312.

26. Walton DM, Macdermid JC, Giorgianni AA, Mascarenhas JC, West SC, Zammit CA. Risk factors for persistent problems following acute whiplash injury: update of a systematic review and meta-analysis. J Orthop Sports Phys Ther 2013;43:31–43.

27. Williamson E, Williams M, Gates S, Lamb SE. A systematic literature review of psychological factors and the development of late whiplash syndrome. Pain 2008;135:20–30.

CHAPTER 14

Manual and Exercise Therapies in Whiplash-Associated Disorders

Alice Kongsted

MANUAL AND EXERCISE THERAPIES

Manual therapy is hands-on techniques aimed at decreasing pain and restoring biomechanical function. The term includes joint manipulation, joint mobilization, and several soft tissue techniques such as massage, trigger point treatment, and stretching techniques. Different manual techniques are often combined in clinical practice. Exercise therapy can be defined as a series of specific movements conducted with the aim of training or developing the body [1]. Different types of exercise therapies aim at different effect mechanisms and include exercises aimed at decreasing pain, increasing muscle strength and endurance, increasing range of motion, normalizing muscle recruitment patterns, and exercises targeting impairments in balance and proprioception. In clinical practice, manual and exercise therapies are often combined and used alongside some level of patient information and advice.

Although there is a theoretical rationale for choosing the type of therapy based on physical impairments, it is only sparsely investigated whether treatment effects are actually mediated through altering the impairments that the therapies are designed to address. There is evidence that impairments in muscle recruitment are improved by exercise therapies [2, 7, 8], but it is not clear whether clinical improvements can be attributed to change in biomechanical function. In low back pain, which to some extent resembles neck pain, most existing evidence does not support that observed effects of exercise therapies are mediated through improved muscular function [13, 17, 23]. Similarly, the effect mechanisms of manual therapies are largely unproven.

MANUAL THERAPY AND EXERCISES AS FIRST-LINE CARE AFTER WHIPLASH EXPOSURE

Treatment Goals and Rationale of Initial Care

Treatments provided in the acute phase after whiplash injuries should give direct symptom relief, but, even more importantly, prevent the development of a chronic pain condition. Mechanisms for the development of chronic whiplash-associated disorders (WAD) are not clear, and a specific diagnosis that could direct treatment choices can generally not be established. However, several factors have been identified that are associated with a poor prognosis after whiplash injuries, and it makes sense to address potentially modifiable prognostic factors in an attempt to prevent chronic WAD. Neck pain intensity and cervical range of motion, which are likely to be positively affected by manual therapy and exercises, are prognostic markers rather consistently found associated with an increased risk of long-lasting WAD [24]. Also, prognostic markers like recovery expectations, fear of movement, catastrophizing, and passive coping strategies may be indirectly affected.

In assessing any treatment effect, it needs to be recognized that single elements of a clinical consultation never work in isolation, and treatment effects result from specific effects of treatment techniques as well as from unspecific effects of the patient–clinician interaction. Clinicians offering manual treatment and exercise therapies often see a patient for a course of treatment, and will potentially affect patients' expectations, beliefs, and fears considerably. This can either be through a conscious attempt to do so or as an undeliberate result of patients' interpretations of information and acts.

Observations of less favorable outcomes with more intense care raise the question of whether health care has iatrogenic effects in acute WAD [5]. It can be hypothesized that offering treatment in the acute phase after a whiplash injury may support an undesirable focus on symptoms or make patients think their acute symptoms are unexpected. On the other hand, it can be speculated that offering care that makes sense to patients will affect patients' beliefs positively and that a course of treatment provides an option to deal with unsolved questions and worrying thoughts. It is unknown to what extent these mechanisms are in play and to what extent patients' expectations and beliefs related to a whiplash injury are actually modifiable. Even with the same care offered, it is most likely that some patients get positive reassurance from the patient–clinician interaction, whereas negative beliefs are reinforced in others. Patients receiving more intensive care do on average have worse outcomes than those with fewer health care visits, but it is not clear whether this is caused by an iatrogenic effect of intensive care or whether the poor prognosis is a result of the factors that made patients seek more care.

Effects of Manual Treatment and Exercise Therapies as First-Line Care

There is no evidence that long-lasting WAD can be effectively prevented by any intervention offered soon after a whiplash injury. Still, the collective research effort does provide some guidance for acute whiplash care.

First of all, the recovery from an acute whiplash injury is not promoted by rest or immobilization. Previously, it was standard care in emergency units to provide patients with a soft neck collar to give pain relief and provide an opportunity for soft tissue sprains to heal. However, evidence consistently shows the absence of a positive effect of advocating rest as treatment in acute WAD. Any type of exercise therapy and also cervical mobilization is more beneficial [21, 22, 26, 27], and immobilization with a soft neck collar may even be harmful [26]. However, from one large trial it seems that prescribing a semirigid collar to severely affected patients apparently does not provide a worse outcome than active strategies [12], and that use of a neck collar for a short period is not likely to be harmful when combined with adequate information. The lack of positive effects from immobilization may be because it actually does not stimulate tissue healing, or because of negative psychological effects, or a combination of the two. In parallel with results in WAD, the results of long-term immobilization as treatment for acute ankle sprains, which was previously standard care, also does appear unfavorable [11]. Like rest and immobilization, also passive physiotherapy modalities such as heat and electrotherapies have been proven ineffective in acute WAD [26].

Since previous standard care including advice to rest was disproven, it is recommended that emergency departments and clinicians seeing patients shortly after a whiplash injury provide information that reinforces a positive prognosis after a whiplash injury and motivates patients to stay active. Whether better outcomes are achieved if advice is standardized and focused on active strategies is still unclear [3, 14, 15, 20], but a large-scale well-conducted trial set up in the United Kingdom did not provide evidence that training emergency department staff to deliver active management strategies made any difference [14].

Although exercise programs, active mobilization, and advice to act as usual in general provide positive effects as compared with rest and passive modalities, it is not clear whether any of these interventions are more effective than others. Also, it is unrevealed whether specific types of exercises are superior to others.

It is possible that the observed lack of impact on the prognosis by early interventions results from a large proportion of patients improving irrespectively of whether they received early treatment or not. Another, potential reason why most interventions appear equally effective is that not all patients need the same kind of care. Stratified care that targets treatments to the individual patient's risk factors or impairments has therefore gained some attention, but it is unknown whether differentiated treatment at the initial visit after a whiplash injury improves outcomes.

Given that treatment effects are not convincing, it could be argued that patients should not be offered care in the acute phase after whiplash injuries. However, patients who are offered minimal care as control interventions in randomized trials (typically, basic advice and analgesics) tend to seek additional care on their own. To avoid excessive doctor shopping and the uncertainties it may lead to if patients have several different explanations for their symptoms and different suggestions about treatment, it therefore seems important that patients consider the first-line care offered adequate.

In sum, which type of care is offered in the very early phase after a whiplash injury has not been proven to make any substantial difference in relation to the risk of developing chronic WAD. Care should be given that avoids rest and immobilization, supports positive expectations, and is considered sufficient by the patient. It should also be recognized that intense treatment plans may have iatrogenic effects.

MANUAL THERAPY AND EXERCISES IN PATIENTS WITH SUSTAINED WAD

Treatment Goals and Rationale

Even when symptoms last, after the first few days a gradual improvement is expected, and interventions in a subacute phase will, to a large extent, still aim at symptom improvement. However, in people who have not achieved acceptable improvement during the first few months after a whiplash injury, manual therapy and exercise interventions will have less focus on pain reduction, and the focus shifts toward restoring function. In patients with severe activity limitations, the aim of these interventions will be to gradually increase physical activity with an emphasis on empowering patients to self-manage their condition.

Patients with long-lasting WAD constitute a heterogeneous group of patients that includes patients with very complex clinical presentations, and the clinical approach will depend on the individual clinical presentation. A range of physical impairments present in chronic WAD such as reduced cervical range of motion, altered movement and muscle recruitment patterns, and signs of altered cervical proprioception can potentially be addressed by manual treatment and exercise therapies. This would suggest specific treatments targeted at such findings. However, many patients with long-lasting pain have very complex presentations that ask for a multifaceted approach in which long-lasting WAD is addressed as a chronic pain condition rather than primarily as a dysfunction of the cervical spine.

Interventions that include manual therapy, exercises, and physical activity are designed to increase patients' physical functioning. However, in addition to such possible specific effects of interventions, it is also likely that psychological factors including fear of movement and depressed mood are affected by treatments that encourage movement and physical activity [4].

Effects of Manual Treatment and Exercise Therapies in Sustained WAD

As for acute WAD, there is no strong evidence to support treatment decisions when symptoms have not resolved. Treatment decisions, therefore, have to be guided also by rationale and evidence from non-traumatic neck pain and from chronic pain conditions in general.

When symptoms do not improve substantially within 3 to 4 weeks, a general clinical approach will be to use treatments directed at the individual patients' symptoms and clinical findings by combining different treatment elements. The documented results of such targeted treatments are mixed.

On the one hand, there is indication that patients who in spite of a thorough initial information return for care after a few weeks with ongoing symptoms, have some additional benefit from treatment combining manual therapy, exercise, advice, and simple psychological strategies matched to the individual risk factor profile as compared with merely reinforcing the initial information [14]. On the other hand, an approach that offered a combination of pharmacotherapy, manual therapy, specific neck exercises, and proprioceptive training guided by the individual factors did not find this superior to usual care in patients with WAD of a maximum duration of 4 weeks; actually, rather the reverse [10]. In the light of the evidence suggesting that too much care early after a whiplash injury may have iatrogenic effects, it could be speculated that the multimodal approach delivered in the last mentioned trial may have been too extensive, since most treatment plans involved visits to different health care professionals, whereas multimodal treatment was delivered in combined sessions in the first mentioned.

In WAD of more than 3 months' duration, it appears highly challenging to design interventions that lead to sustained clinically important effects. A very comprehensive individually tailored exercise program with integrated cognitive–behavioral strategies was not demonstrated to be more effective than one educational session [18]. However, supervised training combined with home exercises has been observed by others to be more effective than advice or prescribing physical activity [16, 25]. At present, it cannot be deduced whether one program of extensive supervised training is truly more effective than another. However, regardless of intervention, a large proportion of patients with long-lasting WAD, unfortunately, do not achieve substantial symptom reduction. Also, in nontraumatic long-lasting neck pain, there is uncertainty about effects of exercise and manual therapy, but supervised exercise sessions appear beneficial [6, 9]. A combination of exercise therapy and manual therapy may yield better results than those obtained from one modality on its own [19], and the goal with manual therapy in long-lasting WAD would often be to achieve symptom relief so that patients are able to be physically active and participate in training activities.

Taken together, the knowledge about treatment effects in subacute WAD, after a few weeks with unresolved symptoms and in long-lasting WAD, may point toward a few weeks with symptoms being a "window of opportunity" in which positive effects are achieved with treatment. This is at the point when fast natural recovery has not occurred and there are still no extensive physiological, psychological, or social consequences of the condition.

A GENERAL APPROACH TO WAD CARE

Although evidence from WAD research does not provide firm answers about optimal care, it does provide guidance for a rational stepwise approach, as outlined in Fig. 14-1.

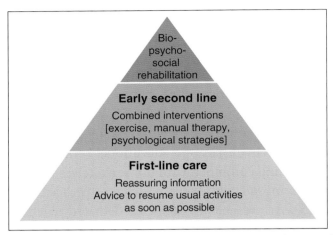

FIGURE 14-1 Intervention triangle illustrating the suggested general approach to WAD interventions. First-line care should be offered to everybody seeking care because of a whiplash exposure. Early second-line care is offered to patients who have not improved adequately within a few weeks after the exposure. Patients developing chronic WAD should be cared for as recommended generally in chronic pain conditions.

First-Line Care

When people seek care shortly after a whiplash trauma and have no fractures or subluxations, the main elements of care are providing reassuring information and advice about avoiding excessive rest and resuming usual activities as soon possible. Initial care should be simple, since nothing is gained in terms of better outcomes by adding more elements to treatment; at the same time, it should be thorough enough to be considered adequate by patients. The initial visit should include a careful examination to rule out serious tissue damage and to help patients rely on reassurance being pertinent in their specific situation. Patients should be informed about WAD, the expected course, and why staying active is encouraged. The personal information should be supported by a leaflet, video, or other educational material that repeats or reinforces the content of the information.

When substantial symptoms persist after 3 to 4 weeks, a course of treatment sessions in which elements of supervised exercises, manual therapy, and simple handling of psychological issues are delivered as one treatment should be considered. There is no strong evidence of effect, but this is probably the best point to initiate treatment to avoid overtreatment of acute patients and yet not adopt a wait-and-see attitude for so long that treatment-resistant chronic symptoms develop.

No convincingly effective treatment exists for patients with long-lasting severe WAD, and interventions in this phase should be considered rehabilitation with a goal of restoring participation in society rather than curing symptoms.

REFERENCES

1. Abenhaim L, Rossignol M, Valat JP, Nordin M, Avouac B, Blotman F, Charlot J, Dreiser RL, Legrand E, Rozenberg S, Vautravers P. The role of activity in the therapeutic management of back pain. Report of the International Paris Task Force on Back Pain. Spine (Phila Pa 1976) 2000;25(4, Suppl):1S–33S.

2. Beer A, Treleaven J, Jull G. Can a functional postural exercise improve performance in the cranio-cervical flexion test?—a preliminary study. Man Ther 2012;17(3):219–24.

3. Brison RJ, Hartling L, Dostaler S, Leger A, Rowe BH, Stiell I, Pickett W. A randomized controlled trial of an educational intervention to prevent the chronic pain of whiplash associated disorders following rear-end motor vehicle collisions. Spine 2005;30(16):1799–807.

4. Cooney GM, Dwan K, Greig CA, Lawlor DA, Rimer J, Waugh FR, McMurdo M, Mead GE. Exercise for depression. Cochrane Database Syst Rev 2013;(9):CD004366.

5. Cote P, Soklaridis S. Does early management of whiplash-associated disorders assist or impede recovery? Spine (Phila Pa 1976) 2011;36(25, Suppl):S275–S279.

6. Evans R, Bronfort G, Schulz C, Maiers M, Bracha Y, Svendsen K, Grimm R, Garvey T, Transfeldt E. Supervised exercise with and without spinal manipulation performs similarly and better than home exercise for chronic neck pain: a randomized controlled trial. Spine (Phila Pa 1976) 2012;37(11):903–14.

7. Falla D, Lindstrom R, Rechter L, Boudreau S, Petzke F. Effectiveness of an 8-week exercise programme on pain and specificity of neck muscle activity in patients with chronic neck pain: a randomized controlled study. Eur J Pain 2013;17(10):1517–28.

8. Falla D, O'Leary S, Farina D, Jull G. The change in deep cervical flexor activity after training is associated with the degree of pain reduction in patients with chronic neck pain. Clin J Pain 2012;28(7):628–34.

9. Gross A, Kay TM, Paquin JP, Blanchette S, Lalonde P, Christie T, Dupont G, Graham N, Burnie SJ, Gelley G, et al. Exercises for mechanical neck disorders. Cochrane Database Syst Rev 2015;(1):CD004250.

10. Jull G, Kenardy J, Hendrikz J, Cohen M, Sterling M. Management of acute whiplash: a randomized controlled trial of multidisciplinary stratified treatments. Pain 2013;154(9):1798–806.

11. Kerkhoffs GM, van den Bekerom M, Elders LA, van Beek PA, Hullegie WA, Bloemers GM, de Heus EM, Loogman MC, Rosenbrand KC, Kuipers T, et al. Diagnosis, treatment and prevention of ankle sprains: an evidence-based clinical guideline. Br J Sports Med 2012;46(12):854–60.

12. Kongsted A, Qerama E, Kasch H, Bendix T, Bach FW, Korsholm L, Jensen TS. Neck collar, "act-as-usual" or active mobilization for whiplash injury? A randomized parallel-group trial. Spine (Phila Pa 1976) 2007;32(6):618–26.

13. Laird RA, Kent P, Keating JL. Modifying patterns of movement in people with low back pain -does it help? A systematic review. BMC Musculoskelet Disord 2012;13:169.

14. Lamb SE, Gates S, Williams MA, Williamson EM, Mt-Isa S, Withers EJ, Castelnuovo E, Smith J, Ashby D, Cooke MW, et al. Emergency department treatments and physiotherapy for acute whiplash: a pragmatic, two-step, randomised controlled trial. Lancet 2013;381(9866):546–56.

15. Lamb SE, Williams MA, Williamson EM, Gates S, Withers EJ, Mt-Isa S, Ashby D, Castelnuovo E, Underwood M, Cooke MW; Managing Injuries of the Neck Trial Group. Managing Injuries of the Neck Trial (MINT): a randomised controlled trial of treatments for whiplash injuries. Health Technol Assess 2012;16(49):iii–iv, 1–141.

16. Ludvigsson ML, Peterson G, O'Leary S, Dedering A, Peolsson A. The effect of neck-specific exercise with, or without a behavioral approach, on pain, disability and self-efficacy in chronic whiplash-associated disorders: a randomized clinical trial. Clin J Pain 2015;31:294–303.

17. Mannion AF, Caporaso F, Pulkovski N, Sprott H. Spine stabilisation exercises in the treatment of chronic low back pain: a good clinical outcome is not associated with improved abdominal muscle function. Eur Spine J 2012;21(7):1301–10.

18. Michaleff ZA, Maher CG, Lin CW, Rebbeck T, Jull G, Latimer J, Connelly L, Sterling M. Comprehensive physiotherapy exercise programme or advice for chronic whiplash (PROMISE): a pragmatic randomised controlled trial. Lancet 2014; 384(9938):133–41.

19. Miller J, Gross A, D'Sylva J, Burnie SJ, Goldsmith CH, Graham N, Haines T, Brønfort G, Hoving JL. Manual therapy and exercise for neck pain: a systematic review. Man Ther 2010;15(4):334–54.

20. Oliveira A, Gevirtz R, Hubbard D. A psycho-educational video used in the emergency department provides effective treatment for whiplash injuries. Spine 2006;31(15): 1652–7.

21. Rosenfeld M, Seferiadis A, Carlsson J, Gunnarsson R. Active intervention in patients with whiplash-associated disorders improves long-term prognosis: a randomized controlled clinical trial. Spine 2003;28(22):2491–8.

22. Schnabel M, Ferrari R, Vassiliou T, Kaluza G. Randomised, controlled outcome study of active mobilisation compared with collar therapy for whiplash injury. Emerg Med J 2004;21(3):306–10.

23. Steiger F, Wirth B, de Bruin ED, Mannion AF. Is a positive clinical outcome after exercise therapy for chronic non-specific low back pain contingent upon a corresponding improvement in the targeted aspect(s) of performance? A systematic review. Eur Spine J 2012;21(4):575–98.

24. Sterling M, Carroll LJ, Kasch H, Kamper SJ, Stemper B. Prognosis after whiplash injury: where to from here? Discussion paper 4. Spine (Phila Pa 1976) 2011;36(25, Suppl):S330–S334.

25. Stewart MJ, Maher CG, Refshauge KM, Herbert RD, Bogduk N, Nicholas M. Advice or exercise for chronic whiplash disorders? Design of a randomized controlled trial. BMC Musculoskelet Disord 2003;4(1):18.

26. Teasell RW, McClure JA, Walton D, Pretty J, Salter K, Meyer M, Sequeira K, Death B. A research synthesis of therapeutic interventions for whiplash-associated disorder (WAD), Part 2: interventions for acute WAD. Pain Res Manag 2010;15(5):295–304.

27. Vassiliou T, Kaluza G, Putzke C, Wulf H, Schnabel M. Physical therapy and active exercises—an adequate treatment for prevention of late whiplash syndrome? Randomized controlled trial in 200 patients. Pain 2006;124(1/2):69–76.

INDEX

Note: Page numbers followed by *f* indicate figures; those followed by *t* indicate tables.